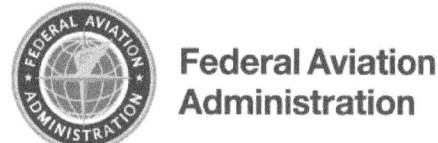 

Federal Aviation Administration

DOT/FAA/AM-07/1
Office of Aerospace Medicine
Washington, DC 20591

Index to FAA Office of Aerospace Medicine Reports: 1961 Through 2006

William E. Collins
CNI Aviation, LLC
Ada, OK 74820

Michael E. Wayda
Civil Aerospace Medical Institute
Federal Aviation Administration
Oklahoma City, OK 73125

January 2007

Final Report

NOTICE

This document is disseminated under the sponsorship of the U.S. Department of Transportation in the interest of information exchange. The United States Government assumes no liability for the contents thereof.

This publication and all Office of Aerospace Medicine technical reports are available in full-text from the Civil Aerospace Medical Institute's publications Web site: www.faa.gov/library/reports/medical/oamtechreports/index.cfm

Technical Report Documentation Page

1. Report No. DOT/FAA/AM-07/1	2. Government Accession No.	3. Recipient's Catalog No.
4. Title and Subtitle Index to FAA Office of Aerospace Medicine Reports: 1961 Through 2006		5. Report Date January 2007
		6. Performing Organization Code
7. Author(s) Collins WE,[1] Wayda ME[2]		8. Performing Organization Report No.
9. Performing Organization Name and Address [1]CNI Aviation, LLC 　　　　[2]FAA Civil Aerospace Medical Institute 2020 Arlington Street　　　　P.O. Box 25082 Ada, OK 74820　　　　　　　Oklahoma City, OK 73125		10. Work Unit No. (TRAIS)
		11. Contract or Grant No.
12. Sponsoring Agency Name and Address Office of Aerospace Medicine Federal Aviation Administration 800 Independence Avenue, S.W. Washington, DC 20591		13. Type of Report and Period Covered
		14. Sponsoring Agency Code
15. Supplemental Notes National Technical Information Service or Defense Technical Information Center order numbers are shown in the chronological listing after the report titles.		
16. Abstract An index to Federal Aviation Administration Office of Aerospace Medicine Reports (1964-2006) and Civil Aeromedical Institute Reports (1961-1963) is presented for those engaged in aviation medicine and related activities. The index lists all FAA aerospace medicine technical reports published from 1961 through 2006: chronologically, alphabetically by author, and alphabetically by subject. A foreword describes the index's sections and explains how to obtain copies of published Office of Aerospace Medicine technical reports. An historical vignette describes some aspects of early toxicological research accomplishments at the Institute.		
17. Key Words Aerospace Medicine, Research Reports, Office of Aerospace Medicine, Civil Aerospace Medical Institute, Civil Aeromedical Research Institute, Human Factors	18. Distribution Statement Document is available to the public through the Defense Technical Information Center, Ft. Belvior, Va. 22060; and the National Technical Information Service, Springfield, VA 22161.	
19. Security Classif. (of this report) Unclassified	20. Security Classif. (of this page) Unclassified	21. No. of Pages 95	22. Price

Form DOT F 1700.7 (8-72)　　　　　　　　　　　　　　　　　　　Reproduction of completed page authorized

Historical Vignette

FIRE AND SMOKE: IMPROVING AVIATION SAFETY THROUGH COMBUSTION TOXICOLOGY RESEARCH

By William E. Collins, Ph.D., and Katherine Wade, M.L.S.

THE HISTORICAL VIGNETTE that follows captures more than two decades of research accomplishments of a biochemistry research team within the Aviation Toxicology Laboratory in the Civil Aeromedical Institute (CAMI). For context purposes, the Toxicology Laboratory (one of several laboratories that originally constituted CAMI's Aeromedical Research Branch) has always comprised a group of research teams identified primarily by their specialty functions. In 2001, CAMI was renamed the Civil Aerospace Medical Institute, and the Toxicology Laboratory became the Bioaeronautical Sciences Research Laboratory.

The vignette represents a self-initiated summarization by Donald Sanders, a research chemist, who developed the material during the 1980s and early 1990s. Its purpose was a means of orienting new laboratory employees on the research activities of Sander's team during the period between 1970-1992. We became aware of the document as a result of publishing a Milestone report of CAMI research in 2005 (DOT/FAA/AM-05/3) when Sanders, who has remained in contact with CAMI personnel since his 1997 retirement, commented that he had prepared some historical material years ago. After reviewing his manuscript, we planned it for inclusion in this issue of the Index, a vehicle previously used to capture historical vignettes, and added some photo documentation.

Donald C. Sanders earned B.S. and M.S. degrees in chemistry from Oklahoma State University and was an instructor there prior to joining CAMI in 1963. His early assignments involved biochemical research on biocidal additives to aircraft fuels (additives that prevented bacterial and fungal growth in the fuel-water interface of the tanks) and issues associated with the exposure of agricultural pilots to the pesticides they used in spraying fields. The latter was an area of particular emphasis in the Toxicology Laboratory during the 1960s. In 1972, Sanders and two long-term associates, John Abbott and Boyd Endecott (both research chemists), began their exploration of combustion toxicology problems in the aviation environment. The team was headed by Charles R. Crane, Ph.D., a biochemist with degrees from the University of Oklahoma (B.S. and M.S.) and Florida State University (Ph.D.). Crane, an assistant professor at Oklahoma State University prior to joining CAMI in 1961, retired in 1988 and was replaced by Arvind K. Chaturvedi in 1990. Chaturvedi obtained his Ph.D. from Lucknow University, India, and had taught at Vanderbilt University and at North Dakota State University.

During the 5-year period from the end of his historical summary to his retirement from federal service, Sanders (along with Endecott, who retired in 2000) remained a part of the new Biochemistry team where he addressed new tasks including drug/altitude effects and aeromedical aspects of melatonin. He also continued his work on combustion toxicology problems with an emphasis on determining coefficients that would allow prediction of time-to-incapacitation for various mixtures of carbon monoxide and hydrocyanic acid — the principal toxic gases produced by fire in aircraft cabins.

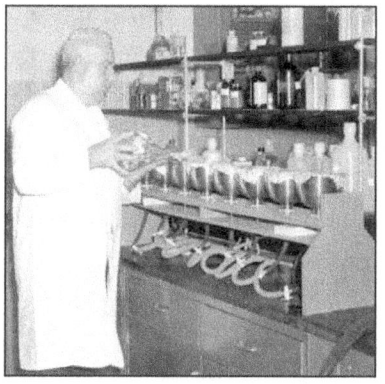

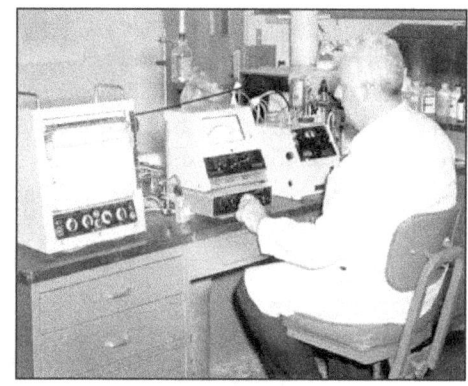

Sander's initial research at CAMI included studies of a biocidal boron-containing additive for aircraft fuels (left) and of plasma-cholinesterase levels in agricultural pilots (crop dusters) exposed to organophosphate pesticides (right).

Combustion Toxicology Research in the Biochemistry Research Unit, CAMI, 1970-1992

By Donald C. Sanders

BACKGROUND

In the early 1960s, aeromedical scientists became aware of the possible significance of smoke toxicity to survival in postcrash aircraft fires. It was observed that some victims with no impact-related physical injuries died as a result of the ensuing fire. The inevitable questions arose as to what killed them, how could this be proven, and how could this risk be reduced or even prevented in future crashes. The Civil Aeromedical Institute's (CAMI's) Forensic Toxicology Unit, within the Aviation Toxicology Laboratory in the Aeromedical Research Branch, found that victims from such fire accidents invariably had elevated blood carboxyhemoglobin (COHb) levels, indicating inhalation of carbon monoxide (CO) from the fire. In early 1969, the Biochemistry Research Section (then a "unit" comprised of Charles Crane, Ph.D., and a staff of Donald Sanders, Boyd Endecott and John Abbott) became interested in the observation that such COHb values ranged from 35 to 85 percent saturation levels. The obvious questions were: What is the minimal lethal COHb value, and, if CO was not responsible for the death of victims below such values, why did they die? Since there was a possibility that some of the reported COHb values might be in error, our first investigation was an evaluation of the analytical techniques commonly used in standard forensic toxicology laboratories. We found that for postmortem analysis under anything less than ideal conditions, the use of the established colorimetric procedures could introduce considerable error. A substitute gas chromatographic technique was therefore recommended.

A PROGRAM OF BASIC STUDIES

CAMI's Biochemistry section became directly involved following an impact-survivable accident at Anchorage, Alaska, in 1970. A Capitol International Airways DC-8 had crashed on takeoff (1), and blood specimens from the victims of the ensuing postcrash fire were found to contain cyanide (2). We then undertook a systematic study of the inhalation of both CO and hydrogen cyanide (HCN), using experimental laboratory animals, to establish some basic relationships for these gases. Although it was now recognized that CO was a probable cause of death in smoke inhalation, the emotional impact of discovering highly toxic **cyanide** in the blood of accident victims affected public opinion enough to require actual research into its origin in aircraft fires.

At that time, little was known about the potential of various aircraft interior components for producing toxic combustion gases in a fire. It was surprising that little documented data existed pertaining to the relative human toxicity of the individual combustion gases themselves. The existing analytical methods, particularly for HCN, lacked specificity, sensitivity and/or reproducibility. Questions regarding the concentrations of CO and HCN produced in aircraft fires and their relationship to the postmortem findings of blood cyanide and carboxyhemoglobin remained essentially unanswered.

Our first animal study was a joint project with Wright-Patterson Air Force Base in Ohio to determine 5-min LC_{50} (a dose lethal to 50% of those exposed) values for CO and HCN and to analyze tissue cyanide levels in rats exposed to these specific concentrations of HCN. The resulting analyses convinced us that the then-current methods for measurement of tissue cyanide were completely inadequate. We therefore modified a gas chromatographic detector (converted a flame ionization detector to a nitrogen-phosphorus detector) and developed a method for HCN determination that exceeded the existing colorimetric, fluorometric, and specific electrode standards for specificity and sensitivity. Research in 1970-1972 was devoted to developing methods for determining CO and HCN in chamber atmospheres and in the blood of exposed animals, developing suitable standards for hemoglobin determination, and studying the effects of blood storage conditions on COHb and cyanide content. During 1973, we further refined our sampling and analytical techniques and looked briefly at rhodanese inhibitors to improve storage stability of HCN in blood and tissue samples.

Finally, in early 1974, we began our first in-house rat exposures to HCN, using a 205-L chamber designed by the section personnel and built in the Civil Aeromedical Institute shop. The chamber employed insert cages for LC_{50} determinations and less conventional, motor-driven rotating cages for the determination of incapacitation. Our approach to the measurement of combustion gas effects differed from that of conventional toxicologists in that we realized that the widely accepted LC_{50} values were of limited application when estimating escape time from a fire environment. We required the definition of the time dependence of the toxic gases on living organisms. We elected to look for the occurrence of psychomotor failure, or physical incapacitation, as our principal endpoint, because that would signal the end of an individual's effective efforts toward unassisted escape from an aircraft. A second deviation from convention was the decision not to count the numbers of rats incapacitated or expired in an arbitrary time period, but to measure the interval between the beginning of exposure and the occurrence of incapacitation or death for each rat (3).

For these initial studies, HCN was generated **in situ** by mechanically injecting a sodium cyanide solution into stirred 10% sulfuric acid inside the chamber. CO exposures were accomplished by injecting commercially available 100% tank CO into the chamber with a 2.8-liter "syringe" of our own construction. By the end of March 1974, we had performed triplicate exposures to CO, to HCN, and to a CO-HCN mixture. These early studies, although crude by today's standards, did serve to justify our choice of a physiological end point; time-to-incapacitation (t_i) occurred at a fraction of the corresponding time-to-death (t_d).

During the following six months, we continuously refined our exposure methodology and analytical techniques, investigated gender-related susceptibility (in rats) to CO and HCN, and performed parallel analyses for HCN by colorimetric and gas chromatographic methods. Two important applications were developed during that period. First, the "dose" for the purpose of defining dose-response relationships in inhalation toxicology, is historically defined as the concentration of the gaseous agent plus an additional parameter, the time over which the exposure takes place. By integrating the area under our concentration-vs-time curves from zero to t_i, we were able to define a "dose," actually a concentration-time product, that was related to a specific t_i. The second application utilized Guyton's relationship of minute-respiratory-volume (MRV) to animal weight in different animal species (4). Assuming that an incapacitating "dose" would be the same for rats of equal weight and that dose, divided by the animal weight, would give us the incapacitating dose per unit of body weight, we developed an equation relating dose, concentration, time, and weight of the animal. Thus, an incapacitating dose, D, could be expressed as $D = [C \bullet t \bullet MRV]/Wt$, where C = concentration in ppm, $t = t_i$, MRV = minute respiratory volume in cm^3/min, and Wt = animal weight in grams (5,6). The equation was equally valid for changing concentrations if the C•t product for the integrated area between zero and t_i were used to replace C and t in the formula. This provided the capability to predict biological responses between species for toxic gases whose mechanism of action was a stoichiometric reaction with critical tissue elements, and hence proportional to total body mass. More pertinent was the exciting possibility of comparing research on nonhuman species to the limited data on human exposures to combustion gases. For CO at least, our calculated physically incapacitating dose for a human, as extrapolated to a 70-kg rat, agreed with the dose predicted by Peterson and Stewart (7) for human acquisition of a 46.5% COHb saturation (8).

A SHIFT TOWARD MATERIALS TESTING

Initially, our research had been directed toward determining basic information about individual combustion gases. The eventual goal was aimed at converting speculative observations into predictive science. Then, in late 1974, the FAA's Office of Aviation Medicine requested that we attempt to assess the relative toxic potential for numerous aircraft interior materials by exposing animals to their pyrolysis products. The request stipulated that the pyrolysis system be similar to one employed at the FAA Technical Center in New Jersey (now the William J. Hughes Technical Center) to allow correlation of our biological findings with the chemical analysis of pyrolysis mixtures to be accomplished by the Technical Center scientists.

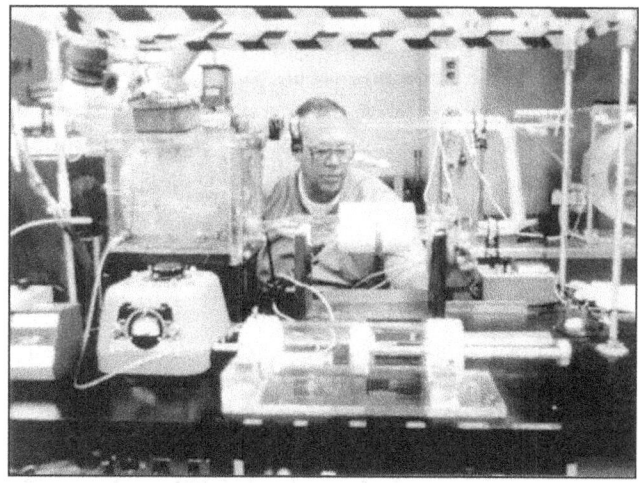

This test exposure by Endecott was performed with CAMI's small, flow-through tubular furnace.

In designing our own system (8), we drew heavily on our previous experience with pure gases. Chamber volume was kept at a minimum to reduce the quantity of sample material needed. The isothermal heating regimen was sufficient to ensure thermal degradation of all organic components in the samples (600°C), and the combustion products were rapidly conducted into the exposure chamber. Oxygen concentration in the chamber was maintained above 90% of ambient, and the temperature was maintained below 35°C. We selected a maximum exposure period of 30 minutes to keep the carbon dioxide concentration below 5% and to minimize the effect of metabolic detoxification on animal response.

Over the course of the year, beginning in mid-1975, we performed triplicate tests on 75 aircraft interior materials and rank-ordered them based on relative t_i and on t_d. We investigated changes in relative rank order when t_i and t_d response times to equal material weights were compared to the orders obtained when rearranged to reflect the **loss** of equal weights during pyrolysis. We also calculated response times corrected for both differences in animal weights and sample weights to define the merits of selecting one system over another for a specific application. We compared different materials within their functional types, i.e., foams, insulations, elastomers, etc. Overall relative standard deviation for the t_i responses for all materials was 13-14%, thus proving the reproducibility of the system for making toxicity measurements of gaseous environments, although the thermal decomposition process did not necessarily represent the actual processes existing in a "real" fire.

Testing the 75 materials proved to be a true learning experience. We had shown (to ourselves, at least) that bioassay could produce very precise endpoints. Deviation from the mean value for 9 rat responses was usually less than 5%, even though individual groups of 3 rats were exposed a month or more apart. It appeared that animals exposed to the same mixture of toxic products on successive occasions reacted the same, and that extreme deviations were related to variations in the combustion process. Materials producing extremely variable results were usually composites, such as layered panels or mixtures of non-uniform composition, that offered sampling difficulties. It was apparent that we had inadequate knowledge about the dynamics of combustion. While we suspected that both the rate of generation and composition of combustion gases would vary with the temperature, oxygen supply, and presence or absence of an ignition source, we had little hard data from the fixed set of conditions imposed on the previous study.

Our next major effort was directed toward developing a new combustion system where sample heating could be programmed, airflow could be controlled over the decomposing sample, and a controllable ignition source could produce flaming or non-flaming combustion as desired. Concurrently, we pursued research to identify the variables of a small-scale test for toxicity. The variables included such diverse factors as effects of carbon dioxide inhalation on breathing rate (and its subsequent effect on t_i when combined with other toxicants), preliminary animal exposures to hydrogen sulfide and sulfur dioxide, and the determination of minimum t_is

from high concentrations of CO and HCN to further refine our equation for the describing t_i-vs-concentration curves. We also developed a smoke detection unit for the combustion system that would record smoke density-vs-time during individual material tests.

In 1977, the Biochemistry Section began a study of the toxic potential of 14 state-of-the-art insulating materials for electrical conductors sponsored by the Urban Mass Transportation Administration (9). These materials were selected from a larger group of insulations being evaluated by the Boeing Commercial Airplane Company for properties other than toxicity. Although we determined rat response per unit weight of insulation, we normalized the data to response per unit length of conductor to permit comparison of insulated conductors on the basis of their intended end use. This study utilized our modified 2-inch diameter combustion tube, wrap-around heating units, and a spark igniter. The system allowed us to investigate differences in animal response times to combustion gases produced during three different heating conditions: 1) low-temperature, nonflaming; 2) low-temperature flaming with hot-wire ignition; and 3) high-temperature, flaming at 750°C with or without ignition. Differences in response times noted at different combustion conditions prompted the proposal that materials should be tested at several conditions and ranked on the "worst case performance" found.

OUR INFLUENCE EXPANDS

During this period (1977-78), section personnel participated in a National Bureau of Standards (NBS) ad hoc committee effort to devise and evaluate a small-scale animal

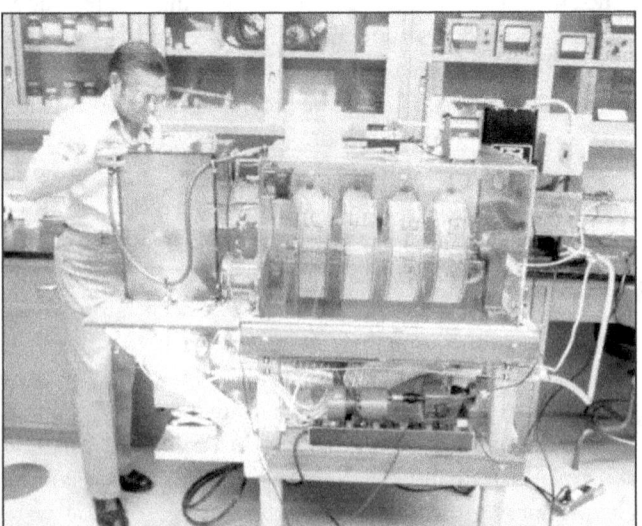

CAMI's large, rotating cage chamber with a "Potts" furnace was used by Crane for this gas exposure test.

test procedure that could be recommended for identifying materials capable of producing "unusually" toxic combustion products. This effort evolved into an inter-laboratory study in which eight different laboratories separately evaluated a control set of standard materials for their combustion toxicity and compared results. Participation in this evaluation required that we modify our 205-L chamber, previously used for pure gas studies, to accommodate a "Potts furnace" combustion unit in an attached chamber, to develop insert chambers for rats that would allow head-only exposure, and to build a "leg-lift" shock avoidance device to measure the specified incapacitation response. The final protocol was adopted in January 1980; our laboratory participation in the cooperative study was concluded in June of that year. The study, although informative, was not conclusive. The published method (10) was used to compare materials on the basis of the toxicity of their combustion products and modification of the method (11) was recommended "for research and preliminary screening purposes."

The ranking of materials by the original method (10) was generally opposed by the plastics industry. It should be remembered that many, if not most, of the researchers who were participating in method development during that period were associated with the wood and plastics industries. Vested interests influenced many of the suggested cut-off levels for determining "unusually toxic" materials; suggestions of "more toxic than the principal product of the company represented" were common. This concern was not entirely unwarranted. A generally accepted test method, perhaps legally enforced, that indicated the superiority of one product over another, could have a devastating effect on manufacturers of the lesser product. Such an outcome would be clearly unfair if the laboratory test method were not (or could not be) validated by corresponding tests in a large-scale fire.

While participating in the NBS cooperative study, we continued to test some state-of-the-art materials that showed promise for use in aircraft interiors and to perform combustion toxicity tests on a variety of materials when requested by outside agencies. These included foam mattress material from a Columbia, Tennessee, jail fire that killed 42 people, Proban-treated wool for the Civil Aviation Attaché to the British Embassy, safety slide material for the American Safety Equipment Company, and rocket propellants for the Thiokol Chemical Corporation. Our research during 1978 was directed toward establishing the thermal tolerance limits of rats and mice subjected to acute exposures at elevated air temperatures. For this limited study, we built a heated and insulated chamber, equipped with a rotating cage assembly, to evaluate the undefined effects of thermal stress on the rats commonly used in combustion toxicology research (12). Dr. Charles Crane also investigated the limited data on human tolerance limits to elevated temperature and proposed rationales for predicting human escape time in rising temperature environments (13) and predicting human tolerance limits to systemic toxic gases (14, 15). Speculative correlations were made between human incapacitation and postmortem COHb/blood cyanide findings in fire-related aircraft accidents (16).

During 1978-1979, Dr. Crane participated in the discussions of the Special Aviation Fire and Explosion Reduction (SAFER) Committee established by the FAA's Flight Standards Service to recommend ways to improve survivability in post-crash environments (17). This committee, and its individual working groups, represented government, industry, and academia. Recommendations for both short- and long-term solutions for post-crash fire hazard reduction and selection of compartment interior materials were extensively discussed.

IRRITANT GAS STUDIES BEGIN

By mid-1980, we began preliminary studies of irritant gas effects. Hydrogen chloride (HCl) gas is a major decomposition product of halogenated polymers such as polyvinyl chloride and polychloroprene used wiring insulation, seats, and fabrics (18). Initial experiments indicated that we would need a high flow rate of HCl gas through the chamber to maintain a fixed concentration due to the extreme solubility of the gas in aqueous (body) fluids. We built a small (12-L) chamber with an enclosed motor-driven rotating cage, adapted a colorimetric method for quantitating gaseous HCl, and determined the t_i and t_d responses by a series of single rat exposures. Individual rat tests were necessary for whole-body exposures because equilibrium concentrations could not be maintained using multiple animals. The HCl (gas) concentrations required to produce incapacitation proved markedly greater than those reported in the scientific literature of that period and suggested that the literature values for humans might have been based on discomfort indices instead of actual incapacitation (18). We were also able to modify another chamber to allow head-only exposures to HCl (gas) in multiples of four rats/test to examine delayed deaths following fixed time/concentration exposures. This chamber also enabled us to remove animals immediately following death for COHb analysis after exposure to CO and to CO-HCl gas mixtures.

Our modest success with the HCl (gas) study encouraged us to consider another irritant gas, acrolein, that had been reported as a combustion product of certain materials used in aircraft interiors. In March through May of 1981, we developed a gas chromatographic method for acrolein determination in air and confirmed it by a separate colorimetric analysis. Rat exposures, in the following two months, indicated that concentrations required to produce incapacitation were also greater than those suggested by the scientific literature; equations were derived from our empirical data to allow prediction of t_i and t_d for the laboratory rat (19). It should be noted that our approach to the study of the biological responses to each of the combustion gases included a quantitative mathematical correlation between concentration and response time. We considered that if combustion toxicology was to become a predictive science, this kind of correlation would allow chemical analysis of smoke with subsequent computer modeling to gradually replace rat exposures as a measure of toxicity.

In mid-1981, several accidents involving turboprop aircraft occurred that were believed to have resulted from pilot incapacitation from toxic fumes introduced through the cabin pressurization system. It was alleged that a broken carbon seal in the engine would allow lubricating oil to enter the air compressor section, allowing oil-contaminated air to enter the cabin and causing a degradation of pilot performance. We initiated a study of the effects of the thermal decomposition products of selected petroleum-based and synthetic lubricating oils. We also examined exposure to aerosols of one synthetic lubricant and of paraffin oil. We found that none of the products generated smoke components significantly more toxic than the quantity of CO produced, which, in the engine tests, was reported to be insignificant (20). It also marked our only experience with the laboratory generation of aerosols for animal exposure studies.

Beginning in late 1981, we were requested by the Transportation Systems Center (TSC) to evaluate the toxicity of the thermal decomposition products from six electrical wiring insulations selected from a group of candidate materials by Factory Mutual Research of Norwood, Massachusetts. Evaluation was by the methods used in the 1977 study (9), and a composite ranking for these and the 14 materials in the earlier study was prepared at the request of the TSC technical monitor (21). One additional "halogen-free" wiring insulation was also tested using this method.

The wiring insulation study took up most of the section's activity in 1982. Between material testing sessions, we evaluated soot penetration into the respiratory system of the rat when exposed to smoke from burning polyvinyl chloride pipe. We also found that rats with artificial nasal obstructions were incapacitated by HCl in about half the time required for control rats. A preliminary look at species differences was obtained by exposures of gerbils to CO and to the gases from a modacrylic fabric (a known CO and HCN producer).

Another inhalation toxicology related problem was investigated in 1982 at the request of the Office of Aviation Medicine. The use of dry ice as pellets or powdered forms instead of the previously used block form caused concern about the relative rates of sublimation inside cargo aircraft. Dry ice shipments were believed to pose a particular hazard aboard smaller transport aircraft, where the pressurized cargo and personnel compartments are combined. Using the controlled temperature and humidity chambers of the CAMI Protection and Survival Laboratory, we performed a limited study to relate sublimation rates to dry ice from packaging, temperature, and humidity, and related them to the equation in Advisory Circular AC 103-4 for calculating the maximum allowable weight of dry ice cargo (22).

In 1983, we installed a radiant heat assembly in the combustion plenum of a 205-L chamber to allow us to thermally decompose flat materials (such as panels), using a unidirectional heat application; this would allow multilayered materials to decompose in a sequential manner such as they might in a real fire scenario. A recirculation system was developed to allow airflow around the sample, both to supply oxygen to the burning material and to prevent smoke buildup (with subsequent loss of radiant heat flux at the sample position). Using sample sizes scaled down to the 12.6-L chamber size, we compared rat response times and gas concentration/time curves in the two chambers, thus examining the feasibility for further scale-up to something nearer a real-fire situation. Beginning in October of 1983, we performed extensive toxicity tests on two aircraft seat fire-blocking materials designed to delay the involvement of thermally sensitive polyurethane foam seat cushions in an aircraft fire. Each material was decomposed by unidirectional (radiant heat) and omnidirectional (combustion tube) heat in five distinct thermal environments. Sample size was expressed on the basis of surface area per system volume to equate both the end use function of the materials and the difference in volumes of the test systems (23).

Additional material testing took up most of the Biochemistry section's activity in 1984. In March, we performed combustion tests on 4 wiring insulation samples at the request of the New York City Transit Authority. In June, we began toxicity tests on 9 panels that were concurrently being evaluated for flammability and smoke production at the FAA Technical Center using their C-133 aircraft cabin test assembly. These panels were tested using both flaming and nonflaming conditions, 12.6-L vs 265-L chambers, and unidirectional radiant heat vs omnidirectional radiant and conductive heat (combustion tube). The shortest t_is (i.e., worst case condition) occurred at the highest temperature/heat flux condition for both chambers (24). Late in 1984, we built an additional radiant heat assembly for use with the combustion tube/small chamber unit to enable us to compare tests in the two systems using similar methods of thermal decomposition.

During this period, the FAA reviewed the possibility that passenger protective breathing devices could be designed for commercial aircraft that would provide some degree of passenger protection from smoke/combustion products and still be compatible with the decompression protective systems in current use. Dr. Crane summarized CAMI's related combustion toxicology research and its application to the problem of survival in inflight aircraft fires in a panel presentation at the 1984 Aerospace Medical Association's annual scientific sessions (25).

A LOOK AT INTERACTIVE EFFECTS

In 1985, we attempted to measure the changes in frequency and amplitude of respiration in the rat with increasing atmospheric carbon dioxide concentrations. With the somewhat crude equipment available, we were able to measure frequency of respiration in an unrestrained rat, but rat movement and cage motion in the rotating cage system prevented integration of the signal to obtain the actual minute respiratory volume. A rat restraining tube, designed for head-only rat exposure, was equipped with an outlet to a pressure transducer, but even the minimal animal movement within the restrainer prevented accurate integration of the respiratory volume with time. The head-only exposure insert restrainer did allow us to study the effects of CO exposures at an elevated chamber temperature (60°C) without raising the animal's core temperature and to measure the corresponding COHb levels at death. We found no statistical difference in the measured parameters between exposures at room temperature and at 60°C.

In late 1985, we acquired a commercial animal exposure chamber containing a rotating "drum" that rotated toward a shock platform; in it, a single rat was required to walk atop the drum to avoid an electrical shock. Early 1986 was spent in fitting the chamber with a flow-through system for introducing gas-air mixtures, in evaluating animal incapacitation in terms of the shock avoidance response, and in adapting a tetracyanonickelate method for the determination of gaseous HCN. These extensive preparations were directed toward a detailed reexamination of the combined effects of CO and HCN on the laboratory rat, a study interrupted some ten years earlier by the agency's material testing requirements. Exposures to CO, HCN, and to mixtures of the two gases occupied the remainder of 1986. Results indicated that the toxic potencies of the two gases were fractionally additive, with no indication of synergism. Dose-response modeling,

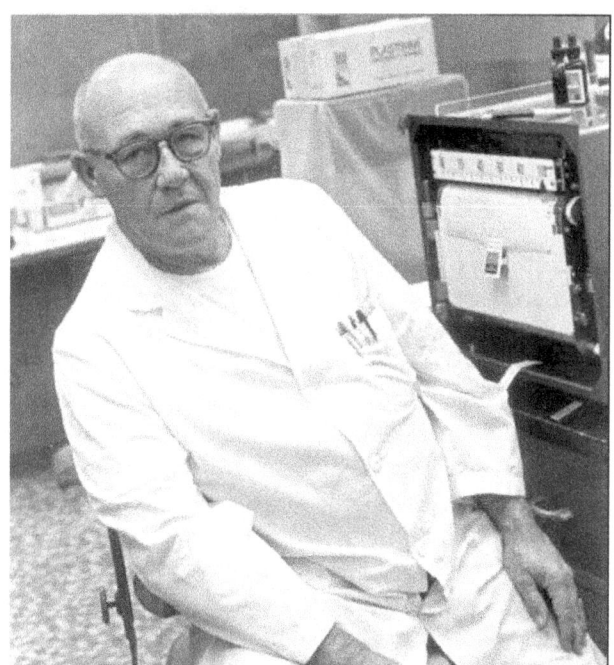

Abbott at the team's gas chromatograph used to measure carbon monoxide concentrations in the rat exposure chamber.

based on the concept of "fractional effective doses," was used to devise a mathematical model for estimating t_i produced by defined mixtures of CO and HCN (26). Some material testing continued during this period including a fire-resistant foam produced by Polyvoltac, Canada, and some multi-layer panels manufactured by Schneller, Inc. of Kent, Ohio.

Formal requests for material testing were becoming fewer by 1987, allowing us time to plan experiments that would expand our understanding of the effects of different basic combustion parameters such as gas mixtures, heat, and changes in the pyrolysis process itself. Industry and government were beginning to understand that the ranking of materials on the basis of their potential fire toxicity was a very complex problem and that some of the early approaches to its solution had been overly simplistic. Not enough was known about the combined effects of individual combustion gases to warrant toxicity predictions from the chemical analysis of combustion products, and even with animal models, no laboratory test for fire toxicity of materials had been validated by an equivalent large-scale test model.

One of the unanswered questions involved what the quantitative effect of an irritant gas such as HCl or acrolein might be on the toxicity of the systemic toxicants, CO and HCN. In mid-1987, we began our first rat exposures to CO, acrolein, and CO-acrolein mixtures. We found evidence of an "antagonistic like" effect when acrolein was present in the CO-acrolein mixture at a concentration less toxic than that of the CO, that is, the t_i was longer than would have been predicted for the CO concentration alone. When the toxic potency of acrolein in the mixture exceeded that of the CO, t_i began to decrease as the acrolein ceased to act simply as a respiration-depressing irritant and began to exert its own toxic effects. Regression equations were developed to predict t_i for the rat when exposed to known concentrations of CO and acrolein, singly and in mixtures (27,28).

The acquisition of a mass flow-controller allowed us to establish a dynamic flow system in an exposure chamber that allowed direct placement of an experimental animal inside the rotating cage after concentration equilibrium had been established. This eliminated the problems of exposing the rat to a changing gas concentration during initial buildup or decay and relating an average concentration to the observed response. A high flow rate through the chamber eliminated any concentration drop at animal insertion. With this modification, we examined the variation in rats' t_i responses to CO at concentrations that produced nominal 5-, 10-, and 25-min t_is; corresponding relative standard deviations were 3, 10, and 19%. This enabled us to refine our CO response equation using more rigidly controlled concentration values.

Some limited material testing continued in 1987. Three panel materials proposed for use in passenger aircraft interiors were tested at the request of the Phillips 66 Company and the Boeing Commercial Airplane Company. Rankings were based on equal surface areas of the sample specimens, again in consideration for their end-use applications (29). We also tested three foam cushion materials at the request of Chestnut Ridge Foam, Inc., one of which had been evaluated as a potential seat blocking material by the FAA Technical Center. Although these tests did not represent any official acceptance or rejection of the foams (no official test criteria existed), copies of the memorandum report of our results, appropriately highlighted and labeled, were distributed by the company as promotional material at a national sales meeting (30). Certain manufacturers and users of the foams used for comparison in the study (which were not manufactured by Chestnut Ridge Foam, Inc.) were not pleased with the use of the report. That venture caused us to consider carefully any future requests for testing of manufacturer-supplied sample materials.

SETBACKS ... AND REJUVENATED SUPPORT

In January of 1988, Dr. Charles Crane retired, having been with CAMI since its inception in 1961. His leadership of the Biochemistry Research Section, particularly after the applied research trends directed our efforts toward combustion toxicology, was characterized by a willingness to start with very basic concepts and thus lay the groundwork for the logical progression to applicable knowledge. He was a perfectionist, who believed that any analytical method accepted for use should be checked by at least one other independent method. His approach to combustion toxicology was not that of the conventional toxicologist; he insisted that animal responses be numerically equated with defined gaseous or thermal insults and that the "dose-response" relationships be mathematically modeled to make combustion toxicology a predictive rather than a purely descriptive science. In short, he brought a sense of logic and order to a research field noted for its self-serving and emotional biases.

A significant administrative crisis in the Aeromedical Research Branch led to limited funds for the entire Aviation Toxicology Laboratory in 1988; we were allotted zero equipment money and only $800 for supplies for the year and were now reduced to two researchers, Donald Sanders and Boyd Endecott. John Abbott had previously retired in January 1986. With technical advice from CAMI's Protection and Survival Laboratory personnel, we modified an existing animal exposure chamber to provide a controlled thermal environment and a stable, flow-through CO-air atmosphere. With this equipment, we investigated the effect of moderately elevated, whole-body temperatures on the rat's t_i response to fixed concentrations of CO. Equations were derived from the data to describe the t_i relationships to temperature and CO concentrations, both singly and when simultaneously applied. The fractionally additive incapacitating effects reaffirmed the necessity for temperature control when the rat is used for combustion gas testing (31,32).

In 1989, we studied the relative toxic hazard rankings of identical materials by t_i and by LC_{50}, the principal indices used to measure the toxicity of combustion products. Pure polymeric standards were selected to provide uniformity of sample composition and to allow selection of a broad range of probable gas compositions; combustion conditions were identical for all tests. Relative rankings by the two endpoints were not identical. We found that delayed deaths were possible, even when incapacitation did not occur during the acute exposure and that LC_{50} values give little indication of available escape time in a fire environment. An additional determination of t_is at the experimentally determined LC_{50} values gave a broad range of values for the same set of polymers at this defined condition of equal lethality (33).

Initial plans for 1990 research were to identify the concentrations of CO and HCN that would produce incapacitation in the laboratory rat at 5 and 35 min and to expose a sufficient number of animals to each fixed concentration to determine the variation in the t_i response. This information had been requested for use by a Society of Automotive

Engineers Aviation Working Group that was involved in defining international standards for passenger protective breathing equipment and in which one of the section scientists (Donald Sanders) had previously participated. After Arvind K. Chaturvedi, Ph.D., joined the Biochemistry Research section as supervisor in January 1990, as part of a rejuvenation of support for the entire laboratory, the project was extended to include the measurements of COHb and blood cyanide at t_i. Intermediate experimental results indicated the desirability of determining uptake kinetics for relating blood concentrations with chamber gas concentrations and time. Results indicated that blood concentrations were both time- and concentration-dependent and that no fixed concentration of either blood cyanide or COHb corresponded to the onset of the incapacitation response. The cyanide uptake was essentially linear, and an equation was developed to predict blood cyanide levels in the rat for known exposure times and concentrations. A limited study of rats exposed to CO-HCN mixtures indicated that any effect on individual gas uptake by the second gas in the mixture was minimal (34,35).

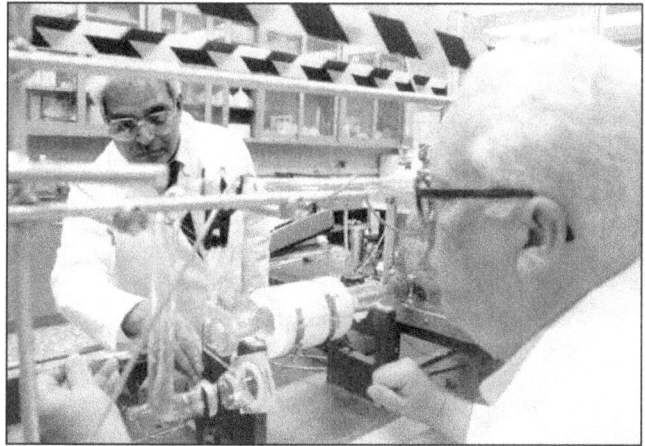

Chaturvedi (left) and Sanders combine efforts in setting up the team's small, flow-through combustion assembly.

A SUMMARY OF ACCOMPLISHMENTS

Often in science, what seem to be definitive answers lead to new questions, which lead to new answers, and the cycle goes on. So what did we really accomplish in over 22 years (1970-1992)? Summarizing the preceding chronological record, we developed mathematical relationships from experimental data equating concentrations of the principal combustion gases of importance in civil aviation with t_i using the rat model. For the systemic toxicants, we demonstrated that the dose-response relationships derived from animal studies can be used to calculate dose-response relationships for humans, provided the proper scaling factors are used. Because real fires generate multiple combustion products, we investigated the effects of simultaneous inhalation of two systemic toxicants (CO-HCN) and of a systemic toxicant paired with an irritant gas (CO-acrolein) and developed empirical equations to predict t_i (in the rat) from the relative concentrations of these gases in mixtures. Finally, we quantitatively described the combined effects of elevated temperature and CO concentration on the t_i response in the rat model.

In material testing studies, we investigated different methods of pyrolysis in an attempt to match pyrolysis conditions to a probable condition in a real fire environment. We noted the effects of changes in the burning conditions on the generation rate, composition, and concentration of the resulting combustion gases. Concurrently, we also investigated the specific gases produced, both by chemical analyses and by their biological effects, and compared a variety of physiological endpoints for measuring the relative toxic potencies of polymer combustion products. It became apparent that, whatever testing system was used to rank materials for combustion toxicity, materials must be compared on a quantitative basis related to their end use, i.e., foams by equal volume, panels by equal surface area, wiring insulations by equivalent length of conductor, etc. It was also apparent that all materials needed to be tested in their final formulations, including all coloring materials, fire retardants, and surface coatings, since each of these could (and frequently did) contribute to the toxicity of the resulting combustion gases.

Throughout the studies, we attempted to define each factor in the material combustion/exposure/response relationships in such a way that the information gained could be used to sequentially refine the conditions for succeeding experiments. This stepwise approach also allowed us to mathematically reevaluate data from older studies in the light of our newer findings. The in-house construction of most of the animal exposure chambers, and their subsequent operation, made us painfully aware of their original design shortcomings and allowed us to innovatively improve them to increase the precision of replication in animal exposures.

Perhaps overshadowing these contributions to combustion toxicology are advances that remain to be accomplished. Even today, state-of-the-art combustion toxicology has no generally accepted standard method for ranking materials on the basis of the relative toxicity of their combustion products. There is no "standard" fire condition, nor are there any small-scale laboratory test methods, adequately validated by comparable full-scale fire tests, that will reliably rank competing candidate materials to reflect their overall fire hazard. Regrettably, there has been little, if any, reduction in the use of rats for toxicity testing. Although we developed the products that government requested (and industry frequently resisted), there proved to be few simplistic answers to the abundance of complex problems.

UNFINISHED BUSINESS

Based on our years of experimental research studies, what remains to be done before we can ever hope to meaningfully assess the potential fire hazard of materials by laboratory testing and subsequent mathematical modeling? In the area of material combustion, we must mathematically define the effects of heating rates, types of ignition and amounts of available oxygen on the rate of production, composition, and concentration of combustion products. Any laboratory-scale "test" must be validated by parallel large-scale tests that directly compare defined loads of test materials. In animal testing, it would be desirable to measure the actual uptake of the toxicants, not time-concentration measurements, and to equate these actual doses with specific physiological end points. This would enable us to make judgments on an actual dose-per-unit-weight basis, which would enhance the application of rat data to the human model. We need to examine the actual mechanisms of action for each toxicant on the living organism and its systems and to determine effects of multiple toxicants on the relative uptake of each. Fire-generated aerosols still remain a relatively unexplored problem. How are they generated and what are their biological effects? Accurate mathematical modeling will depend on the quantitative interpretation of each of these cause-effect relationships. Even if the combustion products are of an exposure that does not produce incapacitation or death, what are the long-term health risks that result?

Many of the questions related to the effects of combustion conditions and individual material screening can probably be answered by approaches utilizing a combination of engineering and bioanalytical chemistry techniques. Limited animal testing may still be required to look for the occasional "supertoxic" material that might not be detected in a screening test for expected combustion gases. We also need to remind ourselves that potential fire toxicity is only one problem in the selection of the "safest" materials for aircraft interiors. Material properties such as flammability, tensile strength, durability, cost, and amount of the specific material used, must also be considered if meaningful judgments are to be made. If the material doesn't burn, then smoke toxicity isn't a problem! What we probably should **not** do is require that material selection be regulated solely on the basis of existing, small-scale toxicity tests, which are neither sophisticated nor reliable enough to accurately evaluate acute and long-term toxic hazards for humans.

REFERENCES

1. National Transportation Safety Board, Aircraft Accident Report: Capitol International Airways, Inc. DC-8-63F, N4909C, Anchorage, Alaska, November 27, 1970, Report No. NTSB-AAR-72-12, File No. 1-0025, 1972.

2. Smith, P.W., C.R. Crane, D.C. Sanders, J.K. Abbott, and B.R. Endecott. FAA Studies of the Toxicity of Products of Combustion. Applied Physics Laboratory/Johns Hopkins Report No. APL/JHU FPP B 76-1, April 1976.

3. Smith, P.W. and C.R. Crane. Biological Testing in Fire Toxicology. Presentation at 3rd Joint Meeting of U.S.-Japan Panel on Fire Research and Safety, Washington, D.C., March 13-17, 1978.

4. Guyton, A.C. Measurement of the Respiratory Volumes of Laboratory Animals. Am J Physiol, 150:70-7, 1947.

5. Sanders, D.C., C.R. Crane, P.W. Smith, J.K. Abbott, and B.R. Endecott. Effects of Exposure to Carbon Monoxide and Hydrogen Cyanide. Presented at the Annual Scientific Meeting of the Aerospace Medical Association, San Francisco, CA, April 28-May 1, 1975.

6. Crane, C.R. The Prediction of Human Incapacitation by the Combustion Products Carbon Monoxide and Hydrogen Cyanide Using a Small Animal Test Protocol. Presented at the Annual Scientific Meeting of the Aerospace Medical Association, Washington, D.C., May 14-17, 1979.

7. Peterson, J.E. and R.D. Stewart. Human Absorption of Carbon Monoxide from High Concentrations in Air Am Ind Hyg Assoc J, 33:293-7, 1972.

8. Crane, C.R., D.C. Sanders, B.R. Endecott, J.K. Abbott, and P.W. Smith. Inhalation Toxicology: I. Design of a Small Animal System, II. Determination of the Relative Toxic Hazards of 75 Aircraft Cabin Materials. FAA report No. FAA-AM-77/9, March 1977.

9. Crane, C.R., B.R. Endecott, D.C. Sanders, and J.K. Abbott. Electrical Insulation Fire Characteristics. Vol. II: Toxicity. U.S. Department of Transportation, Urban Mass Transportation Administration Report No. UMTA-MA-06-0025-79/2, II., March 1979.

10. Birky, M.M., M. Paabo, B.C. Levin, S.E. Womble, and D. Malek. Development of Recommended Test Method for Toxicological Assessment of Inhaled Combustion Products. NBSIR 80-2077, Washington, D.C., National Bureau of Standards, 1980.

11. Levin, B.C., A.J. Fowell, M.M. Birky, M. Paabo, A. Stolte, and D. Malelz. Further Development of a Test Method for the Assessment of the Acute Inhalation Toxicity of Combustion Products. NBSIR 82-2h 2532, Washington, D.C., National Bureau of Standards, 1982.

12. Crane, C.R. and D.C. Sanders. Inhalation Toxicology: VIII: Establishing Heat Tolerance Limits for Rats and Mice Subjected to Acute Exposures at Elevated Air Temperatures. FAA Report No. DOT/FAA/AM-86/8, May 1986.

13. Crane, C.R. Human Tolerance Limits to Systemic Toxic Gases. FAA Memorandum Report No. AAC-114-78-1, April 14, 1978.

14. Crane, C.R. Human Tolerance Limit to Elevated Temperature: An Empirical Approach to the Dynamics of Acute Thermal Collapse. FAA Memorandum Report No. AAC-114-78-2, May 5, 1978.

15. Crane, C.R. The Prediction of Human Incapacitation by the Combustion Products Carbon Monoxide and Hydrogen Cyanide Using a Small Animal Test Protocol. Presented at the Annual Scientific Meeting of the Aerospace Medical Association, Washington, D.C., May 14-17, 1979.

16. Kirkham, W.R., D.J. Lacefield, and C.R. Crane. Toxicological and Pathological Findings in Aircraft Accident Victims that Indicate Incapacitation from Burning Interior Materials. Presented at the Annual Scientific Meeting of the Aerospace Medical Association, Washington, D.C., May 14-17, 1979.

17. Ferrarese, J.A. Establishment and Invitation to Participate: Special Aviation Fire and Explosion Reduction (SAFER). Federal Register, Vol. 43, No. 111, June 8, 1978.

18. Crane, C.R., D.C. Sanders, B.R. Endecott, and J.K. Abbott. Inhalation Toxicology: IV. Times to Incapacitation and Death for Rats Exposed Continuously to Atmospheric Hydrogen Chloride Gas. FAA Report No. FAA-AM-85/4, May 1985.

19. Crane, C.R., D.C. Sanders, B.R. Endecott, and J.K. Abbott. Inhalation Toxicology: VII. Times to Incapacitation and Death for Rats Exposed Continuously to Atmospheric Acrolein Vapor. FAA Report No. DOT/FAA/AM-86/5, May 1986.

20. Crane, C.R., D.C. Sanders, B.R. Endecott, and J.K. Abbott. Inhalation Toxicology: III. Evaluation of Thermal Degradation Products from Aircraft and Automobile Engine Oils, Aircraft Hydraulic Fluid, and Mineral Oil. FAA Report No. FAA-AM-83/12, April 1983.

21. Crane, C.R., D.C. Sanders, B.R. Endecott, and J.K. Abbott. Combustibility of Electrical Wire and Cable for Rail Rapid Transit Systems, Volume II: Toxicity. Urban Mass Transportation Administration Report UMTA-MA-06-0025-83-7, May 1983.

22. Crane, C.R. and D.C. Sanders. Hazard Associated with Sublimation of Solid Carbon Dioxide (Dry Ice) Aboard Aircraft. FAA Memorandum Report No. AAC-114-84-1, March 5, 1984.

23. Sanders, D.C., C.R. Crane, and B.R. Endecott. Inhalation Toxicology: V. Evaluation of Relative Toxicity to Rats of Thermal Decomposition Products from Two Aircraft Seat Fire-Blocking Materials. FAA Report No. DOT/FAA-AM-86/1, November 1985.

24. Crane, C.R., D.C. Sanders, B.R. Endecott, and J.K. Abbott. Inhalation Toxicology: VI. Evaluation of the Relative Toxicity of Thermal Decomposition Products From Nine Aircraft Panel Materials. FAA Report No. DOT/FAA/AM-86/3, February 1986.

25. Crane, C.R. Inflight Aircraft Fires, Toxicological Aspects. Panel presentation at the Aerospace Medical Association Scientific Meeting, San Diego, CA, May 7, 1984.

26. Crane, C.R., D.C. Sanders, and B.R. Endecott. Inhalation Toxicology: IX. Times-to-Incapacitation for Rats Exposed to Carbon Monoxide Alone, to Hydrogen Cyanide Alone, and to Mixtures of Carbon Monoxide and Hydrogen Cyanide. FAA Report No. DOT/FAA/AM-89/4, January 1989.

27. Crane, C.R., D.C. Sanders, and B.R. Endecott. Inhalation Toxicology: X. Times-to-Incapacitation for Rats Exposed Continuously to Carbon Monoxide, Acrolein, and to Carbon Monoxide-Acrolein Mixtures. FAA Report No. DOT/FAA/AM-90/15, December 1990.

28. Crane, C.R., D.C. Sanders, and B.R. Endecott. Incapacitation in the Laboratory Rat Induced by Inhalation of Carbon Monoxide-Acrolein Mixtures. J Fire Sci, 10(2):133-159, 1992.

29. Crane, C.R. Relative Inhalation Toxicity of Smoke from Three Thermoplastic Polymer Products. FAA Memorandum Report No. AAM-114-87/1, October 1987.

30. Crane, C.R. and D.C. Sanders. Relative Inhalation Toxicity of Smoke From Three Polymeric Foam Products. FAA Memorandum Report No. AAM-114-87/2, December 1987.

31. Sanders, D.C. and B.R. Endecott. Inhalation Toxicology: XI. The Effect of Elevated Temperature on Carbon Monoxide Toxicity. FAA Report No. DOT/FAA/AM-90/16, December 1990.

32. Sanders, D.C. and B.R. Endecott. The Effect of Elevated Temperature on Carbon Monoxide-Induced Incapacitation. J. of Fire Sciences 9(4):296-310, 1991, and in Advances in Combustion Toxicology, Vol. 3, Gordon E. Hartzell, ed., Technomic Publishing Company, Inc., Lancaster, PA, pp. 343-57, 1992.

33. Sanders, D.C., B.R. Endecott, and A.K. Chaturvedi. Inhalation Toxicology: XII. Comparison of Toxicity Rankings of Six Polymers by Lethality and by Incapacitation in Rats. FAA Report No. DOT/FAA/AM-91/17, December 1991.

34. Sanders, D.C., B.R. Endecott, and A.K. Chaturvedi. Variation of Times-to-Incapacitation (t_is) and Carboxyhemoglobin (COHb) Levels for Rats Exposed to Two Carbon Monoxide (CO) Concentrations. Presented at the Annual Scientific Meeting of the Aerospace Medical Association, Miami Beach, FL, May 10-14, 1992.

35. Chaturvedi, A.K., B.R. Endecott, R.M. Ritter, and D.C. Sanders. Incapacitation Times (t_is) and Blood Cyanide (CN^-) Levels for Rats Exposed to Hydrogen Cyanide Gas (HCN). Presented at the Annual Scientific Meeting of the American Society for Pharmacology and Experimental Therapeutics, Orlando, FL, August 14-18, 1992.

How to Use the Index

Organization
The Index is organized in three sections:
1. Chronological Index: a cumulative list of all research reports from 1961 through 2006.
2. Author Index: all contributing authors, in alphabetical order.
3. Subject Index: subjects, listed in alphabetical order.

Some examples are:

06-8 Williams KW: Human factors implications of unmanned aircraft accidents: Flight control problems.
Above: This is an entry from the *Chronological Index* of research reports, shown in cumulative sequence.

Xing J -- --04-17, 05-4, 06-2, 06-6, 06-11, 06-15, 06-22
Above: This is an entry from the *Author Index*, which lists all of the research reports prepared by an author or co-author.

Cosmic radiation
...air carrier crew, exposure of, 80-2, 92-2, 00-33, 03-16, 05-14
Above: An example of entries in the *Subject Index;* refers to all reports that pertain to a specific topic.

Report Numbers
05-2 Corbett CL: Caring for precious cargo, Part II: Behavioral techniques for emergency aircraft evacuations with infants through the Type III overwing exit. ADA460057

Above: The first numbers (05-2) refer to the year and chronological number of the report. This is an abbreviated portion of the official number given each report and is found in the upper left of the report's cover page. The full report number of "05-2" is DOT/FAA/AM-05/2. The "ADA460057" is appended to the report by the National Technical Information Service. Keep the number system in mind when ordering from NTIS.

How to Order or Obtain for Free
- You may purchase copies of OAM Reports from: National Technical Information Service
  Refer to the "ADA" (or other prefixes) 5285 Port Royal Road
  and numbers. Springfield, VA 22161
  Telephone (800) 553-6530

- **The Federal Depository Library System.** Some 1,300 U.S. libraries maintain a reference repository of official Government reports printed by the U.S. Government Printing Office. The reports are either in printed or microform for public use. These libraries provide reference services and interlibrary loans; however, they are not sales outlets.

- Abstracts and full text of all reports are available on the Federal Aviation Administration's Internet site:
  www.faa.gov/library/reports/medical/oamtechreports/index.cfm

- Abstracts and full text of many reports are available from the Defense Technical Information Center's Public STINET Internet site: http://stinet.dtic.mil

- A limited number of back issues are maintained by the Institute. Some requests may be filled by writing to:
  FAA Civil Aerospace Medical Institute
  Aerospace Medical Education Division, AAM-400
  P.O. Box 25082, Shipping Clerk
  Oklahoma City, OK 73125-5064

"Aviation Safety Through the Development and Application of Aeromedical Knowledge."

Contents

Part I
Chronological Index -- 1

Part II
Author Index -- 41

Part III
Subject Index --- 51

PART I: CHRONOLOGICAL INDEX
1961 Through 2006

1961

61-1   Trites DK: Problems in air traffic management: I. Longitudinal prediction of effectiveness of air traffic controllers. AD268954

1962

62-1   Swearingen JJ, Wheelwright CD, Garner JD: An analysis of sitting areas and pressures of man. AD271138

62-2   Cobb BB Jr: Problems in air traffic management: II. Prediction of success in air traffic controller school. N62-10354

62-3   Trites DK, Cobb BB Jr: Problems in air traffic management: III. Implications of age for training and job performance of air traffic controllers. N62-10353

62-4   Swearingen JJ, Mohler SR: Sonotropic effects of commercial air transport sound on birds. AD280212

62-5   Iampietro PF, Goldman R: Prediction of energy cost of treadmill work. AD280607

62-6   Balke B: Human tolerances. AD421156

62-7   Hasbrook AH, Earley JC: Failure of rearward-facing seat backs and resulting injuries in a survivable transport accident. AD421157

62-8   Smith PW: Toxic hazards in aerial application. AD421158

62-9   Hasbrook AH, Garner JD, Snow CC: Evacuation pattern analysis of a survivable commercial aircraft crash. AD282893

62-10   Daugherty JW, Lacey DE, Korty P: Problems in aerial application: I. Some biochemical effects of lindane and dieldrin on vertebrates. AD288413

62-11   Hawkes GR: Tactile communication. AD288414

62-12   Dille JR, Newton NL, Culver JF: The effects of simulated altitude on penetrating eye injuries. AD288415

62-13   Swearingen JJ, Hasbrook AH, Snyder R G, McFadden EB: Kinematic behavior of the human body during deceleration. AD283938

62-14   Swearingen JJ: Determination of centers of gravity of man. AD287156

62-15   Gogel WC: The visual perception of size and distance. AD287197

62-16   Hawkes GR: Absolute identifications of cutaneous stimuli varying in both intensity level and duration. AD295134

62-17   Collins WE: Manipulation of arousal and its effects on human vestibular nystagmus induced by caloric irrigation and angular accelerations. AD290348

62-18   Hinshaw LB, Brake CM, Iampietro PF, Emerson TE Jr: Effect of increased venous pressure on renal hemodynamics. AD295137

62-19   Snyder RG: A case of survival of extreme vertical impact in seated position. AD295136

62-20   Mohler SR: Civil aeromedical research: Responsibilities, aims, and accomplishments. AD295135

62-21   McFadden EB, Raeke JW, Young JW: An improved method for determining the efficiency of crew and passenger oxygen masks. AD297835

1963

63-1   Emerson TE Jr, Hinshaw LB, Brake CM, Iampietro PF: The development of reversible hematuria and oliguria following elevation of renal venous pressure. AD299775

63-2   Mohler SR, Dille JR: Resume and index of reports of the Civil Aeromedical Research Institute, 1961-1962. AD431924

63-3   Collins WE: Observations on the elicitation of secondary and inverted primary nystagmus from the cat by unilateral caloric irrigation. AD413456

63-4   Daugherty JW, Lacey DE, Korty P: Problems in aerial application: II. Effects of chlorinated hydrocarbons on substratelinked phosphorylation. AD418504

63-5   Melton CE Jr: Neural control of the ciliary muscle. AD413392

63-6   Balke B: A simple field test for the assessment of physical fitness. AD413393

Part I: Chronological Index

63-7 Tobias JV, Jeffress LA: Relation of earphone transient response to measurement of onset-duration. AD413391

63-8 McKenzie JM, Fowler PR, Lyne PJ: Calibration of an electronic counter and pulse height analyzer for plotting erythrocyte volume spectra. AD425598

63-9 Swearingen JJ, McFadden EB: Studies of air loads on man. AD602207

63-10 Gogel WC: The perception of depth from binocular disparity. AD429827

63-11 Lategola MT: In vivo measurement of total gas pressure in mammalian tissue. AD425537

63-12 Nagle FJ, Balke B, Ganslen RV, Davis AW: The mitigation of physical fatigue with Spartase. AD429001

63-13 Collins WE: Primary, secondary, and caloric nystagmus of the cat following habituation to rotation. AD428756

63-14 Collins WE: Nystagmus responses of the cat to rotation and to directionally equivalent and nonequivalent stimuli after unilateral caloric habituation. AD425565

63-15 Snyder RG: Human survivability of extreme impacts in free-fall. AD425412

63-16 Emerson TE Jr, Brake CM, Hinshaw LB: Mechanisms of action of the insecticide endrin. AD431299

63-17 Tobias JV: Application of a "relative" procedure to a problem in binaural beat perception. AD428899

63-18 Balke B: Experimental evaluation of work capacity as related to chronological and physiological aging. AD431301

63-19 Wernick JS, Tobias JV: A central factor in pure tone auditory fatigue. AD428737

63-20 Gogel WC: The visual perception of spatial extent. AD432587

63-21 Tang PC, Dille JR: In-flight loss of consciousness: A case report. AD430394

63-22 Hinshaw LB, Page BB, Brake CM, Emerson TE Jr, Masucci FD: The mechanisms of intrarenal hemodynamic changes following acute arterial occlusion. AD431302

63-23 Higgins EA, Iampietro PF, Adams T, Holmes DD: The effects of a tranquilizer on body temperature. AD432484

63-24 Dille JR, Smith PW: Central nervous system effects of chronic exposure to organophosphate insecticides. AD434090

63-25 Adams T, Funkhouser GE, Kendall WW: A method for the measurement of physiologic evaporative water loss. AD603418

63-26 Reins DA, Holmes DD, Hinshaw LB: Acute and chronic effects of the insecticide endrin on renal function and renal hemodynamics. AD602206

63-27 Dille JR, Crane CR, Pendergrass GE: The flammability of lip, face, and hair preparations in the presence of 100% oxygen. AD602204

63-28 Gogel WC: Size cues and the adjacency principle. AD602205

63-29 Collins WE: Task-control of arousal and the effects of repeated unidirectional angular acceleration on human vestibular responses. AD603419

63-30 Snyder RG, Ice J, Duncan JC, Hyde AS, Leverett S Jr: Biomedical research studies in acceleration. AD601531 Supplement-AD801793

63-31 Trites DK, Cobb BB Jr: Problems in air traffic management: IV. Comparison of preemployment, job-related experience with aptitude tests as predictors of training and job performance of air traffic control specialists. AD603416

63-32 Hinshaw LB, Emerson TE Jr, Brake CM: Mechanism of autoregulation in the intact kidney. AD603417

63-33 Dill DB, Robinson S, Balke B, Newton JL: Work tolerance: Age and altitude. AD603932

63-34 Ganslen RV, Balke B, Phillips EE, Nagle F: Effects of some tranquilizing, analeptic, and vasodilating drugs on physical work capacity and orthostatic tolerance. AD603930

63-35 Pearson RG: Human factors aspects of lightplane safety. AD603931

Tech. Pub. #1 Collins WE, Tobias JV, Capps MJ, Allen ME: Annotated bibliography of recently translated material. I. AD424640

1964

64-1 Wentz AE: Studies on aging in aviation personnel. AD456652

64-2 Naughton J, Balke B, Nagle F: The effect of physical conditioning on an individual before and after suffering a myocardial infarction. AD456653

64-3   Nagle FJ, Balke M: The gradational step test for assessing cardiorespiratory capacity: An experimental evaluation of treadmill and step test procedures. AD456654

64-4   Spieth W: Cardiovascular health status, age, and psychological performance. AD453578

64-5   Moser KM: Current status of clot dissolution therapy. AD453579

64-6   Seipel JH, Wentz AE: Unsuspected neurologic disease in aviation personnel: Survival following seizures in flight. AD453580

64-7   Houk VN, Hufnagel CA, McClenathan JE, Moser KM: Chronic thrombotic obstruction of major pulmonary arteries. AD453581

64-8   Moser KM, Perry RB, Luchsinger PC: Cardiopulmonary consequences of pyrogen-induced hyperpyrexia in man.

64-9   Freud SL: Duration of spiral aftereffect as a function of retinal size, retinal place, and hemiretinal transfer. AD618588

64-10 Freud SL: Duration as a measure of the spiral aftereffect. AD618589

64-11 Pinkerson AL, Kot PA, Knowlan DM: Effect of glyceryl trinitrate on pulmonary vasculature of anesthetized dogs.
       64-12 Scarborough WR: Comments on progress in ballistocardiographic research and the current state of the art. AD455651

64-13 Gogel WC: The size cue to visually perceived distance. AD456655

64-14 Capps MJ, Collins WE: Effects of bilateral caloric habituation on nystagmus responses of the cat. AD455652

64-15 Collins WE, Huffman HW: Design and performance characteristics of a mechanically driven vestibular stimulator. AD456656

64-16 Tobias JV, Collins WE, Allen ME: Aviation medicine translations: Annotated bibliography of recently translated material. II. AD456670

64-17 Freud SL: The physiological locus of the spiral aftereffect. AD611881

64-18 Melton CE Jr: Physiological recordings from pilots operating an aircraft simulator. AD456671

64-19 Perloff JK: The recognition of strictly posterior myocardial infarction by conventional scalar electrocardiography. AD611882

64-20 FAA Aviation Medical Library: Aviation medical papers and reports: a bibliography. AD613364

1965

65-1   Capps MJ, Collins WE: Auditory fatigue: Influence of mental factors. AD459636

65-2   Collins WE, Capps MJ: Effects of several mental tasks on auditory fatigue. AD459637

65-3   Reighard, HL: Medical services at airports. AD611883

65-4   Seipel JH, Ziemnowicz SAR, O'Doherty DS: Cranial impedance plethysmography-Rheoencephalography as a method of detection of cerebrovascular disease. AD611884

65-5   Hauty GT, Trites DK, Berkley WJ: Biomedical survey of ATC facilities: I. Incidence of self-reported symptoms. AD689806

65-6   Hauty GT, Trites DK, Berkley WJ: Biomedical survey of ATC facilities: II. Experience and age. N66-16669

65-7   Mohler SR, Swearingen JJ, McFadden EB, Garner JD: Human factors of emergency evacuation. AD459638

65-8   Van Brummelen AGW, Scarborough WR, Josenhans WKT: On the elimination of pulse wave velocity in stroke volume determination from the ultralow frequency displacement ballistocardiogram. AD612450

65-9   Lowenstein 0, Feinberg R, Loewenfeld I: Pupillary movements during acute and chronic fatigue. AD612451

65-10 O'Connor WF, Pearson RG: ATC system error and appraisal of controller proficiency. N66-16583

65-11 Gogel WC: The equidistance tendency and its consequences: Problems in depth perception. AD621432

65-12 Snyder RG: Survival of high-velocity free-falls in water. AD621021

65-13 Mohler SR: Fatigue in aviation activities. AD620022

65-14 Snow CC, Hasbrook AH: The angle of shoulder slope in normal males as a factor in shoulder-harness design. AD653920

65-15 Scarborough WR (Joint NASA-FAA publication): Ballistocardiography: a bibliography N65-35520

65-16 Hauty GT, Adams T: Pilot fatigue: Intercontinental jet flight: Oklahoma City-Tokyo. AD621433

Part I: Chronological Index

65-17 Allen ME, Collins WE, Tobias JV, Crain RA: Aviation medicine translations: Annotated bibliography of recently translated material. III. AD617090

65-18 Collins WE: Adaptation to vestibular disorientation: I. Vertigo and nystagmus following repeated clinical stimulation. AD617091

65-19 Cobb BB Jr: Problems in air traffic management: V. Identification and potential of aptitude test measures for selection of tower air traffic controller trainees. AD620722

65-20 Swearingen JJ: Tolerances of the human face to crash impact. AD621434

65-21 Trites DK: Problems in air traffic management: VI. Interaction of training-entry age with intellectual and personality characteristics of air traffic control specialists. AD620721

65-22 Trites DK, Miller MC, Cobb BB Jr: Problems in air traffic management. VII. Job and training performance of air traffic control specialists-measurement, structure, and prediction. AD649292

65-23 Swearingen JJ, Young JW: Determination of centers of gravity of children, sitting and standing. AD661865

65-24 Collins WE: Adaptation to vestibular disorientation. II. Nystagmus and vertigo following high-velocity angular accelerations. AD621435

65-25 Feinberg R, Podolak E: Latency of pupillary reflex to light stimulation and its relationship to aging. AD689809

65-26 Snow CC, Snyder RG: Anthropometry of air traffic control trainees. N66-25185

65-27 Brake CM, Reins D, Wittmers LE, Hinshaw LB: Intrarenal hemodynamic changes following acute partial renal arterial occlusion. AD649263

65-28 Hauty GT, Adams T: Phase shifts of the human circadian system and performance deficit during the periods of transition: I, East-West flight. AD639637

65-29 Hauty GT, Adams T: Phase shifts of the human circadian system and performance deficit during the periods of transition: II. West-East flight. AD689811

65-30 Hauty GT, Adams T: Phase shifts of the human circadian system and performance deficit during the periods of transition: III. North-South flight. AD689812

65-31 Pearson RG, Hunter CE, Neal GL: Development and evaluation of a radar air traffic control research task. AD660198

65-32 Gogel WC, Mertens HW: Problems in depth perception: A method of simulating objects moving in depth. AD660171

1966

66-1 Allen ME, Mohler SR: Aviation medicine reports: An annotated catalog of Office of Aviation Medicine reports: 1961 through 1965. AD638732

66-2 Allen ME, Crain RA: Aviation medicine translations: Annotated bibliography of recently translated material. IV. AD651907

66-3 Mohler SR, Swearingen JJ: Cockpit design for impact survival. AD687411

66-4 Tobias JV: A table of intensity increments. AD642113

66-5 Clark G: Problems in aerial application: A comparison of the effects of dieldrin poisoning in cold-adapted and room-temperature mammals. N66-30197

66-6 Fiorica V: Fatigue and stress studies: An improved semiautomated procedure for fluorometric determination of plasma catecholamines. AD653748

66-7 McFadden EB: Evaluation of the physiological protective efficiency of a new prototype disposable passenger oxygen mask. AD644118

66-8 Mohler SR: The predominant causes of crashes and recommended therapy. AD639779

66-9 Young JW: Selected facial measurements of children for oxygen mask design. AD640062

66-10 O'Connor WF, Pendergrass GE: Effects of decompression on operator performance. AD675774

66-11 Hinshaw LB, Reins DA, Emerson TE Jr, Rieger JA Jr, Stavinoha WB, Fiorica V, Solomon LA, Holmes DD: Problems in aerial application: I.-V. AD660199

66-12 Swearingen JJ: Injury potentials of light-aircraft instrument panels. AD642114

66-13	McFadden EB, Simpson JM: Flotation characteristics of aircraft-passenger seat cushions. AD642349
66-14	Iampietro PF, Fiorica V, Dille JR, Higgins EA, Funkhouser G, Moses R: Problems in aviation personnel: Influence of a tranquilizer on temperature regulation in man. AD638733
66-15	O'Connor WF, Scow J, Pendergrass GE: Hypoxia and performance decrement. AD639780
66-16	Lategola MT, Harrison HF, Barnard C: The aeromedical assessment of human systolic and diastolic blood-pressure transients without direct arterial puncture. AD639615
66-17	Naughton J, Shanbour K, Armstrong R, McCoy J, Lategola MT: Problems in aeromedical certification: Cardiovascular responses to exercise following myocardial infarction. AD640970
66-18	Swearingen JJ: Evaluation of head and face injury potential of current airline seats during crash decelerations. AD653869
66-19	Pearson RG: Performance tasks for operator-skills research. AD642115
66-20	McFadden EB, Lategola MT: Evaluation of the Sierra hanging quick-don crew pressure-breathing oxygen mask. AD645493
66-21	Naughton J, Lategola MT, Shanbour K: Clinical aviation medicine: A physical-conditioning program for cardiac patients. AD640969
66-22	Gogel WC, Mertens HW: Problems in depth perception: Perceived size and distance of familiar objects. AD641477
66-23	Iampietro PF, Adams T: The achievement of thermal balance and its maintenance during environmental stress. AD642350
66-24	Agee FL Jr, Gogel WC: Problems in depth perception: Equidistance judgments in the vicinity of a binocular illusion. AD641476
66-25	Mohler SR, Freud SL, Veregge JE, Umberger EL: Physician flight accidents. AD648768
66-26	Clark G: Problems in aerial application: Histochemistry of Weil stain on liver. AD652599
66-27	Dille JR, Morris Edward W: Human factors in general aviation accidents. AD640971
66-28	Mohler SR: Oxygen in general aviation. AD645497
66-29	Mohler SR: Recent findings on the impairment of airmanship by alcohol. AD644119
66-30	Mohler SR, Harper CR: Protecting the Ag pilot. AD641478
66-31	Von Rosenberg CW, Keen FR, Mohler SR: The "stall barrier" as a new preventive in general aviation accidents. AD642351
66-32	Mohler SR, Hasbrook AH: In-flight response to a new non-gyroscopic blind flight instrument. AD641479
66-33	Young JW: Recommendations for shoulder restraint installation in general aviation aircraft. AD646054
66-34	Clark G: Problems in aerial application: A comparison of the acute effects of endrin and carbon tetrachloride on the livers of rats and of the residual effects one month after poisoning. AD645494
66-35	Melton CE Jr, Wicks SM: Pilot vision considerations: The effect of age on binocular fusion time. AD645495
66-36	Nagle FJ, Naughton J, Balke B: Clinical aviation medicine research: Comparison of simultaneous measurements of intra-aortic and auscultatory blood pressure with pressure-flow dynamics during rest and exercise. AD645496
66-37	Collins WE: Adaptation to vestibular disorientation. III. Influence on adaptation of interrupting nystagmic eye movements with opposing stimuli. AD649615
66-38	Mertens HW: A homogeneous field for light adaptation.
66-39	Melton CE Jr, Higgins EA, Saldivar JT, Wicks SM: Exposure of men to intermittent photic stimulation under simulated IFR conditions. AD646872
66-40	Swearingen JJ: Evaluation of various padding materials for crash protection. AD647048
66-41	McKenzie JM, Fiorica V: Physiological responses of pilots to severe-weather flying. AD646871
66-42	Garner JD, Blethrow JG: Emergency evacuation tests of a crashed L-1649. AD645423

1967

67-1	Cobb BB Jr: The relationships between chronological age, length of experience, and job performance ratings of air route traffic control specialists. AD661468

67-2   Mertens RA, Collins WE: Adaptation to vestibular disorientation. IV. Responses to angular acceleration and to bilateral caloric stimulation following unilateral caloric habituation. AD653696

67-3   McFadden EB: Development of techniques for evaluating the physiological protective efficiency of civil aviation oxygen equipment. AD659498

67-4   McFadden EB, Reynolds HI, Funkhouser GE: A protective passenger smoke hood. AD657436

67-5   Fowler PR, McKenzie JM: Problems in aerial application: Detection of mild poisoning by organophosphorus pesticides using an automated method for cholinesterase activity. AD656211

67-6   Collins WE, Guedry FE Jr: Adaptation to vestibular disorientation. V. Eye-movement and subjective turning responses to two durations of angular acceleration. N67-38956

67-7   Guedry FE Jr, Collins WE: Adaptation to vestibular disorientation. VI. Eye-movement and subjective turning responses to varied durations of angular acceleration. AD671855

67-8   Lewis MF, Ashby FK: Diagnostic tests of color-defective vision: Annotated bibliography, 1956-1966. AD660200

67-9   McFadden EB, Harrison HF, Simpson JM: Performance characteristics of constant-flow phase dilution oxygen mask designs for general aviation. AD660201

67-10 Rowland RC Jr, Tobias JV: Interaural intensity difference limen. AD661235

67-11 Seipel JH: The biophysical basis and clinical applications of rheoencephalography. AD673082

67-12 Collins WE: Adaptation to vestibular disorientation. VII. Special effects of brief periods of visual fixation on nystagmus and sensations of turning. AD659192

67-13 Young JW: A functional comparison of basic restraint systems. AD660202

67-14 Swearingen JJ: An evaluation of potential decompression hazards in small pressurized aircraft. AD660203

67-15 Melton CE Jr, Wicks SM: In-flight physiological monitoring of student pilots. AD665660

67-16 Lewis MF: Cross-modality matching of loudness to brightness for flashes of varying luminance and duration. AD664463

67-17 Funkhouser GE, Billings SM: A portable device for the measurement of evaporative water loss. AD664465

67-18 Gogel WC: Cue-enhancement as a function of task-set. AD664466

67-19 Collins WE: Adaptation to vestibular disorientation. VIII. "Coriolis" vestibular stimulation and the influence of different visual surrounds. N68-16799

67-20 Gogel WC, Mertens HW: Perceived depth between familiar objects. AD665293

67-21 Crane CR, Sanders DC: Evaluation of a biocidal turbine-fuel-additive. AD665661

67-22 Mohler SR, Bedell RHS, Ross A, Veregge EJ: Aircraft accidents by older persons. AD663688

67-23 Veregge EJ: Type airman certification as related to accidents. AD663688

67-24 Lewis MF, Mertens HW: Reaction time as a function of flash luminance and duration. AD664464

67-25 Siegel PV: Aviation medicine, FAA-1966. AD675943

1968

68-1   Index to FAA Office of Aviation Medicine Reports: 1961 through 1967. AD673666

68-2   Collins WE: Adaptation to vestibular disorientation: IX. Influence of head position on the habituation of vertical nystagmus. AD677460

68-3   Podolak E, Kinn JB, Westura EE: Biomedical applications of a commercial capacitance transducer. AD683292

68-4   Fiorica V, Burr MJ, Moses R: Contribution of activity to the circadian rhythm in excretion of magnesium and calcium. AD674416

68-5   Booze CF Jr: Usage of combined airman certification by active airmen: An active airman population estimate. AD678947

68-6   Crosby WM, Snyder RG, Snow CC, Hanson PG: Impact injuries in pregnancy. I. Experimental studies. AD674861

68-7   Allen ME, Mertens RA: Aviation medicine translations: Annotated bibliography of recently translated material. V. AD673665

68-8   Mohler SR, Dille JR, Gibbons HL: Circadian rhythms and the effects of long-distance flights. AD672898

68-9   Siegel PV, Booze CF Jr: A retrospective analysis of aeromedical certification denial actions. January 1961-December 1967. AD675521

68-10 Collins WE, Schroeder DJ: The spiral aftereffect: Influence of stimulus size and viewing distance on the duration of illusory motion. AD673644

68-11 Hasbrook AH, Young PE: Pilot response to peripheral vision cues during instrument flying tasks. AD684804

68-12 Hasbrook AH, Young PE: Peripheral vision cues: Their effect on pilot performance during instrument landing approaches and recoveries from unusual attitudes. AD683305

68-13 Vaughan JA, Higgins EA, Funkhouser GE, Galerston EM: The effects of body thermal state on manual performance. AD675522

68-14 Cobb BB Jr: A comparative study of air traffic trainee aptitude-test measures involving Navy, Marine Corps, and FAA controllers. AD686669

68-15 Higgins EA, Davis AW Jr, Fiorica V, Iampietro PF, Vaughan JA, Funkhouser GE: Effects of two antihistamine containing compounds upon performance at three altitudes. AD676502

68-16 Dille JR, Mohler SR: Drug and toxic hazards in general aviation. AD686670

68-17 Thackray RI, Pearson DW: The effects of cognitive appraisal of stress on heart rate and task performance. AD687413

68-18 Higgins EA, Davis AW Jr, Vaughan JA, Funkhouser GE, Galerston EM: The effects of alcohol at three simulated aircraft cabin conditions. AD686671

68-19 Snyder RG, Snow CC: Fatal injuries resulting from extreme water impact. AD688424

68-20 Lewis MF: Two-flash thresholds as a function of flash luminance and area. AD686672

68-21 Tobias JV: Cockpit noise intensity: Fifteen single-engine light aircraft. AD686425

68-22 Hasbrook AH: A comparison of effects of peripheral vision cues on pilot performance during instrument flight in dissimilar aircraft simulators. AD688425

68-23 Fiorica V: A table for converting pH to hydrogen ion concentration [H+] over the range 5-9. AD688120

68-24 Snyder RG, Snow CC, Crosby WM, Hanson P, Fineg J, Chandler R: Impact injury to the pregnant female and fetus in lap belt restraint. AD689359

68-25 Tobias JV: Cockpit noise intensity: Eleven twin-engine light aircraft. AD688111

68-26 Melton CE Jr, Wicks M, Saldivar JT, Morgan J, Vance FP: Physiological studies on air tanker pilots flying forest fire retardant missions. AD690090

68-27 Lewis MF, Mertens HW: Assessment of the Broca-Sulzer phenomenon via inter- and intra-modality matching procedures: Studies of signal-light brightness. AD689358

68-28 Collins WE: Adaptation to vestibular disorientation. X. Modification of vestibular nystagmus and "vertigo" by means of visual stimulation. AD691405

1969

69-1   Melton CE Jr, Wicks M: Binocular fusion time in sleep-deprived subjects. AD688426

69-2   Siegel PV, Mohler SR: Medical factors in U.S. general aviation accidents. AD689740

69-3   Snyder RG, Snow CC, Young JW, Crosby WM, Price GT: Pathology of trauma attributed to restraint systems in crash impacts. AD690415

69-4   Snyder RG, Young JW, Snow CC: Experimental impact protection with advanced restraint systems: Preliminary primate tests with air bag and inertia reel/inverted-Y yoke torso harness. AD695416

69-5   Snyder RG, Crosby WM, Snow CC, Young JW, Hanson PG: Seat belt injuries in impact. AD698298

69-6   Chiles WD, Bruni CB, Lewis RA: Methodology in the assessment of complex human performance: The effects of signal rate on monitoring a dynamic process. AD697943

69-7   Pearson DW, Thackray RI: Consistency of performance change and autonomic response as a function of expressed attitude toward a specific stress situation. AD697944

69-8   Thackray RI: Patterns of physiological activity accompanying performance on a perceptual-motor task. AD697945

69-9   Chiles WD, Gibbons HL, Smith PW: Effects of two common medications on complex performance. AD703631

Part I: Chronological Index

69-10   Iampietro PF, Chiles WD, Higgins EA, Gibbons HL, Jennings AE, Vaughan JA: Complex performance during exposure to high temperatures. AD703632

69-11   Booze CF Jr: Occupations of active airmen. AD704474

69-12   Melton CE Jr, Hoffmann SM, Delafield RH: The use of a tranquilizer (chlordiazepoxide) in flight training. AD703221

69-13   Snyder RG, Snow CC, Young JW, Price GT, Hanson PG: Experimental comparison of trauma in lateral (+Gy), rearward-facing (+Gx), and forward-facing (-Gx) body orientations when restrained by lap belt only. AD707185

69-14   Chiles WD, Jennings AE: Effects of alcohol on complex performance. AD703633

69-15   Williams MJ, Collins WE: The spiral aftereffect. II. Some influences of visual angle and retinal speed on the duration and intensity of illusory motion. AD703634

69-16   Chiles WD, Bruni CB, Lewis RA: Methodology in the assessment of complex performance: The effects of signal rate on monitoring a static process. AD703635

69-17   Siegel PV, Gerathewohl SJ, Mohler SR: Time-zone effects on the long-distance air traveler. AD702443

69-18   Siegel PV, Mohler SR, Cierebiej A: The safety significance of aircraft accident post mortem findings. AD704473

69-19   Pearson DW, Clark G, Moore CM: A comparison of the behavioral effects of various levels of chronic disulfoton poisoning. AD704470

69-20   Collins WE, Updegraff BP: Adaptation to vestibular disorientation. XI. The influence of specific and nonspecific gravireceptors on nystagmic responses to angular acceleration. AD704471

69-21   Thackray RI, Touchstone RM: Recovery of motor performance following startle. AD704472

69-22   Swearingen JJ, Badgley JM, Braden GE, Wallace TF: Determination of centers of gravity of infants. AD708514

69-23   Brecher MH, Brecher GA: Motor effects from visually induced disorientation in man. AD708425

69-24   Gerathewohl SJ: Fidelity of simulation and transfer of training: A review of the problem. AD706744

1970

70-1   Index to FAA Office of Aviation Medicine Reports: 1961 through 1969. AD714027

70-2   Brecher MH, Brecher GA: Quantitative evaluation of optically induced disorientation. AD709329

70-3   Ryan LC, Endecott BR, Hanneman GD, Smith PW: Effects of an organophosphorus pesticide on reproduction in the rat. AD709327

70-4   Crane CR, Sanders DC, Abbott JK: Studies on the storage stability of human blood cholinesterases: I. AD714028

70-5   Higgins EA, Vaughan JA, Funkhouser GE: Blood alcohol concentrations as affected by combinations of alcoholic beverage dosages and altitudes. AD709328

70-6   Tobias JV: Auditory processing for speech intelligibility improvement. AD717394

70-7   Hasbrook AH, Rasmussen PG: Pilot heart rate during in-flight simulated instrument approaches in a general aviation aircraft. AD711268

70-8   Fiorica V, Higgins EA, Lategola MT, Davis AW Jr, Iampietro PF: Physiological responses of men during sleep deprivation. AD713590

70-9   Gerathewohl SJ, Morris Everett W, Sirkis JA: Anti-collision lights for the supersonic transport (SST). AD713488

70-10   Collins WE, Schroeder DJ, Rice N, Mertens RA, Kranz G: Some characteristics of optokinetic eye-movement patterns: A comparative study. AD715440

70-11   Revzin AM: Some acute and chronic effects of endrin on the brain. AD715452

70-12   Mohler SR: Physiologically tolerable decompression profiles for supersonic transport type certification. AD713055

70-13   Crane CR, Sanders DC, Abbott JK: A comparison of three serum cholinesterase methods. AD715439

70-14   Karson S, O'Dell JW: Performance ratings and personality factors in radar controllers. AD715247

70-15   Lewis MF, Mertens, HW: Two-flash thresholds as a function of comparison stimulus duration. AD716645

70-16   Snow CC, Carroll JJ, Allgood MA: Survival in emergency escape from passenger aircraft. AD735388

70-17   Collins WE: Effective approaches to disorientation familiarization for aviation personnel. AD719003

70-18 Lategola MT, Fiorica V, Booze CF Jr, Folk ED: Comparison of status variables among accident and nonaccident airmen from the active airman population. AD722148

70-19 Garner JD, Blethrow JG: Evacuation tests from an SST mockup. AD720627

70-20 McFadden EB, Smith RC: Protective smoke hood studies. AD727021

70-21 Lategola MT, Harrison HF: A device and method for rapid indirect measurement of human systolic and diastolic blood pressures. AD722032

70-22 Iampietro PF: Tolerances to thermal extremes in aerospace activities. AD722001

1971

71-1 Tobias JV: Noise audiometry. AD723464

71-2 Melton CE Jr, McKenzie JM, Polis BD, Funkhouser GE, Iampietro PF: Physiological responses in air traffic control personnel: O'Hare Tower. AD723465

71-3 Swearingen JJ: General aviation structures directly responsible for trauma in crash decelerations. AD728728

71-4 Iampietro PF: Use of skin temperature to predict tolerance to thermal environments. AD723466

71-5 Mertens RA, Goulden DR, Lacy CD, Jones KN: Aviation medicine translations: Annotated bibliography of recently translated material. VI. AD723467

71-6 Schroeder DJ: Alcohol and disorientation-related responses. I. Nystagmus and "vertigo" during caloric and optokinetic stimulation. AD728314

71-7 Thackray RI, Jones KN: Effects of conflicting auditory stimuli on color-word interference and arousal. AD727018

71-8 Lategola MT: Biodynamic evaluation of air traffic control students between 1960-1963. AD726254

71-9 Cierebiej A, Mohler SR, Stedman VG: Physician pilot- in-command flight accidents, 1964 through 1970. AD724286

71-10 Gerathewohl SJ, Mohler SR, Siegel PV: Medical and psychological aspects of mass air transportation. AD726286

71-11 Fiorica V, Burr MJ, Moses R: Effects of low-grade hypoxia on performance in a vigilance situation. AD727019

71-12 Swearingen JJ: Acceptance tests of various upper torso restraints. AD726253

71-13 Swearingen JJ: Tolerances of the human brain to concussion. AD726287

71-14 Smith RC: Assessment of a "stress" response-set in the Composite Mood Adjective Check List. AD727020

71-15 Fiorica V, Moses R: Automated differential fluorometric analysis of norepinephrine and epinephrine in blood plasma and urine. AD729535

71-16 Schroeder DJ: Alcohol and disorientation-related responses. II. Nystagmus and "vertigo" during angular acceleration. AD730629

71-17 Chiles WD, Iampietro PF, Higgins EA, Vaughan JA, West G, Funkhouser GE: Combined effects of altitude and high temperature on complex performance. AD729536

71-18 Gibbons HL, Fromhagen C: Aeromedical transportation and general aviation. AD728315

71-19 Lategola MT: Changes in cardiovascular health parameters over an eight-year interval in an ATC population segment. AD729537

71-20 Collins WE, Gilson RD, Schroeder DJ, Guedry FE Jr: Alcohol and disorientation-related responses. III. Effects of alcohol ingestion on tracking performance during angular acceleration. AD728843

71-21 Smith RC, Melton CE Jr, McKenzie JM: Affect adjective check list assessment of mood variations in air traffic controllers. AD729832

71-22 Brecher MH, Brecher GA: Effect of a moving optical environment on the subjective median. AD728316

71-23 Melton CE Jr, Fiorica V: Physiological responses of low-time private pilots to cross-country flying. AD728317

71-24 Hasbrook AH, Rasmussen PG: Aural glide slope cues: Their effect on pilot performance during in-flight simulated ILS instrument approaches, AD731848

71-25 Norwood GK: The philosophy and limitations of FAA aeromedical standards, policies, and procedures. AD729538

71-26 Friedberg W, Nelson JM: Calibration of the Concorde radiation detection instrument and measurements at SST altitude. AD732789

Part I: Chronological Index

71-27 Lewis MF, Steen JA: Color-defective vision and the recognition of aviation color signal light flashes. AD729539

71-28 Chiles WD, Smith RC: A nonverbal technique for the assessment of general intellectual ability in selection of aviation personnel. AD728844

71-29 Thackray RI, Touchstone RM, Jones KN: The effects of simulated sonic booms on tracking performance and autonomic response. AD729833

71-30 Smith RC, Cobb BB Jr, Collins WE: Attitudes and motivational factors in terminal area air traffic control work. AD730630

71-31 Mehling KD, Collins WE, Schroeder DJ: The spiral aftereffect: III. Some effects of perceived size, retinal size, and retinal speed on the duration of illusory motion. AD729834

71-32 Steen JA, Lewis MF: Color defective vision and day and night recognition of aviation color signal light flashes. AD730631

71-33 Mohler SR, Gerathewohl SJ: Civil aeromedical standards for general-use aerospace transportation vehicles. AD728318

71-34 Gilson RD, Schroeder DJ, Collins WE, Guedry FE Jr: Alcohol and disorientation-related responses. IV. Effects of different alcohol dosages and display illumination on tracking performance during vestibular stimulation. AD729835

71-35 Smith RC: Personality assessment in aviation: An analysis of the item ambiguity characteristics of the 16PF and MMPI. AD736266

71-36 Cobb BB Jr, Lay CD, Bourdet NM: The relationship between chronological age and aptitude test measures of advanced-level air traffic control trainees. AD733830

71-37 McFadden EB, Young JW: Evaluation of an improved flotation device for infants and small children. AD729836

71-38 Norwood GK: Senior aviation medical examiners conducting FAA first-class medical examinations. AD731849

71-39 Hill RJ, Collins WE, Schroeder DJ: Alcohol and disorientation-related responses: V. The influence of alcohol on positional, rotatory, and coriolis vestibular responses over 32-hour periods. AD735389

71-40 Cobb BB Jr: Air traffic aptitude test measures of military and FAA controller trainees. AD737871

71-41 Higgins EA, Fiorica V, Davis HV, Thomas AA: The acute toxicity of brief exposure of HF, HCl, and N02 and HCN singly and in combination with CO. AD735160

71-42 Mertens HW, Lewis MF: Discrimination of short-duration (two-pulse) flashes as a function of signal luminance and method of measurement. AD737872

1972

72-1 Dille JR, Grimm MH: Index to FAA Office of Aviation Medicine Reports: 1961 through 1971. AD742607

72-2 Yanowitch RE, Mohler SR, Nichols EA: The psycho-social reconstruction inventory: A postdictal instrument in aircraft accident investigation. AD738464

72-3 Sirkis JA: The benefits of the use of shoulder harness in general aviation aircraft. AD739943

72-4 Billings CE, Wick RL Jr, Gerke RJ, Chase RC: The effects of alcohol on pilot performance during instrument flight. AD740778

72-5 Chiles WD, Jennings AE, West G: Multiple-task performance as a predictor of the potential of air traffic controller trainees. AD741736

72-6 Lowrey DL, Langston ED, Reed W, Swearingen JJ: Effectiveness of restraint equipment in enclosed areas. AD739944

72-7 Langston ED, Swearingen JJ: Evaluation of a fiberglass instrument glare shield for protection against head injury. AD740732

72-8 Zeiner AR, Brecher GA: Effects of backscatter of brief high-intensity light on physiological responses of instrument-rated pilots and non-pilots. AD744234

72-9 Rasmussen PG, Hasbrook AH: Pilot tracking performance during successive in-flight simulated instrument approaches. AD743392

72-10 McFadden EB: Physiological evaluation of a modified jet transport passenger oxygen mask. AD743422

72-11 Chiles WD, Jennings AE: Effects of alcohol on a problem-solving task. AD743423

72-12 Crane CR, Sanders DC, Abbott JK: A comparison of serum cholinesterase methods: II. AD744866

72-13 Booze CF Jr: Attrition from active airman status during 1970. AD742608

72-14 Thackray RI, Jones KN, Touchstone RM: The color-word interference test and its relation to performance impairment under auditory distraction. AD743424

72-15 Swearingen JJ, Wallace TF, Blethrow JG, Rowlan DE: Crash survival analysis of 16 agricultural aircraft accidents. AD745257

72-16 Jones KN, Goulden DR, Grimm EJ: Aviation medicine translations: Annotated bibliography of recently translated material. VII. AD747125

72-17 Iampietro PF, Melton CE Jr, Higgins EA, Vaughan JA, Hoffman SM, Funkhouser GE, Saldivar JT: High temperature and performance in a flight task simulator. AD746057

72-18 Cobb BB Jr, Mathews JJ: A proposed new test for aptitude screening of air traffic controller applicants. AD746058

72-19 Chiles WD, West G: Residual performance effects of simulated sonic booms introduced during sleep. AD747989

72-20 Lategola MT: The use of simple indicators for detecting potential coronary heart disease susceptibility in the air traffic controller population. AD747990

72-21 Jennings AE, Chiles WD, West G: Methodology in the measurement of complex human performance: Two-dimensional compensatory tracking. AD745259

72-22 Cobb BB Jr, Mathews JJ, Lay CD: A comparative study of female and male air traffic controller trainees. AD751312

72-23 Smith RC: A study of the State-Trait Anxiety Inventory and the assessment of stress under simulated conditions. AD747991

72-24 Smith RC, Hutto GL: Sonic booms and sleep: Affect change as a function of age. AD749277

72-25 Thackray RI, Jones KN, Touchstone RM: Self-estimate of distractibility as related to performance decrement on a task requiring sustained attention. AD751396

72-26 Lategola MT: The use of simple indicators for detecting potential coronary heart disease susceptibility in the third-class airman population. AD749278

72-27 Karim B, Bergey KH, Chandler RF, Hasbrook AH, Purswell JL, Snow CC: A preliminary study of maximal control force capability of female pilots. AD753987

72-28 Mohler SR: G effects on the pilot during aerobatics. AD751397

72-29 Lewis MF, Mertens HW, Steen JA: Behavioral changes from chronic exposure to pesticides used in aerial application: Effects of Phosdrin on the performance of monkeys and pigeons on variable interval reinforcement schedules. AD749893

72-30 Folk ED, Garner JD, Cook EA, Broadhurst JL: GPSS/360 computer models to simulate aircraft passenger emergency evacuation. AD755542

72-31 Tobias JV: Binaural processing of speech in light aircraft. AD753637

72-32 Tobias JV: Auditory effects of noise on air-crew personnel. AD757239

72-33 Cobb BB Jr, Mathews JJ, Nelson PL: Attrition-retention rates of air traffic controller trainees recruited during 1960-1963 and 1968-1970. AD757933

72-34 Schroeder DJ, Gilson RD, Guedry FE, Collins WE: Alcohol and disorientation-related responses. VI. Effects of alcohol on eye movements and tracking performance during laboratory angular accelerations about the yaw and pitch axes. AD766937

72-35 Collins WE, Iampietro PF: Simulated sonic booms and sleep: Effects of repeated booms of 1.0 psf. AD762988

1973

73-1 Braden GE, Reed W, Swearingen JJ: Application of commercial aircraft accident investigation techniques to a railroad derailment. AD764188

73-2 Smith RC: Job attitudes of air traffic controllers: A comparison of three air traffic control specialties. AD763508

73-3 Revzin AM: Subtle changes in brain functions produced by single doses of mevinphos (Phosdrin). AD763509

73-4 Revzin AM: Transient blindness due to the combined effects of mevinphos and atropine. AD763555

73-5 Yanowitch RE, Bergin JM, Yanowitch EA: The aircraft as an instrument of self-destruction. AD763556

Part I: Chronological Index

73-6   Lewis MF: Frequency of anticollision observing responses by solo pilots as a function of traffic density, ATC traffic warnings, and competing behavior. AD763557

73-7   Cobb BB Jr, Nelson PL, Mathews JJ: The relationships of age and ATC experience to job performance rating of terminal area traffic controllers. AD773449

73-8   Booze CF Jr: Prevalence and incidence of disease among airmen medically certified during 1965. AD773544

73-9   Hasbrook AH, Rasmussen PG: In-flight performance of civilian pilots using moving-aircraft and moving-horizon attitude indicators. AD773450

73-10   Lategola MT, Lynn CA, Folk ED, Booze CF Jr, Lyne PJ: Height and weight errors in aeromedical certification data. AD773452

73-11   Thackray RI, Ryander R, Touchstone RM: Sonic boom startle effects: Report of a field study. AD773451

73-12   Lewis MF, Ferraro DP: Flying high: The aeromedical aspects of marihuana. AD775889

73-13   Tobias JV, Irons FM: Reception of distorted speech. AD777564

73-14   Thackray RI, Jones KN, Touchstone RM: Personality and physiological correlates of performance decrement on a monotonous task requiring sustained attention. AD777825

73-15   Smith RC, Melton CE Jr: Susceptibility to anxiety and shift difficulty as determinants of state anxiety in air traffic controllers. AD777565

73-16   Thackray RI, Touchstone RM, Bailey JP: A comparison of the startle effects resulting from exposure to two levels of simulated sonic booms. AD777581

73-17   Schroeder DJ, Collins WE, Elam GW: Effects of secobarbital and d-amphetamine on tracking performance during angular acceleration. AD777582

73-18   Steen JA, Collins WE, Lewis MF: Utility of several clinical tests of color-defective vision in predicting daytime and nighttime performance with the aviation signal light gun. AD777563

73-19   Constant GN, Goulden DR, Grimm EJ: Aviation medicine translations: Annotated bibliography of recently translated material. VIII. AD776136

73-20   Tobias JV, Irons FM: Ear-protector ratings. AD779552

73-21   Melton CE Jr, McKenzie JM, Polis BD, Hoffmann SM, Saldivar JT: Physiological responses in air traffic control personnel: Houston Intercontinental Tower. AD777838

73-22   Melton CE Jr, McKenzie JM, Smith RC, Polis BD, Higgins EA, Hoffmann SM, Funkhouser GE, Saldivar JT: Physiological, biochemical, and psychological responses in air traffic control personnel: Comparison of the 5-day and 2-2-1 shift rotation patterns. AD778214

73-23   Leeper RC, Hasbrook AH, Purswell JL: Study of control force limits for female pilots. AD777839

1974

74-1   Dille JR, Grimm MH: Index to FAA Office of Aviation Medicine Reports: 1961 through 1973. AD779553

74-2   Mathews JJ, Collins WE, Cobb BB: A sex comparison of reasons for attrition of nonjourneyman FAA air traffic controllers. AD780558

74-3   Collins WE: Adaptation to vestibular disorientation. XII. Habituation of vestibular responses: an overview. AD780562

74-4   Young JW, Fisher RG, Price GT, Chandler R F: Experimental trauma of occipital impacts. AD780668

74-5   Booze C, F Jr: Characteristics of medically disqualified airman applicants during calendar year 1971. AD781684

74-6   Lategola MT, Layne PJ: Amplitude/frequency differences in a supine resting single-lead electrocardiogram of normal versus coronary heart diseased males. AD781685

74-7   Mathews JJ, Collins WE, Cobb BB Jr: Job-related attitudes of nonjourneyman FAA air traffic controllers and former controllers: a sex comparison. AD787238

74-8   Cobb BB Jr, Nelson PL: Aircraft-pilot and other pre-employment experience as factors in the selection of air traffic controller trainees. ADA001039

74-9   Thackray RI, Touchstone RM, Bailey JP: Behavioral, autonomic, and subjective reactions to low- and moderate-level sonic booms: A report of two experiments and a general evaluation of sonic boom startle effects. ADA002266

74-10   Chiles WD, West G: Multiple-task performance as a predictor of the potential of air traffic controller trainees: A follow-up study. ADA002920

74-11   Melton CE Jr, McKenzie JM, Saldivar JT, Hoffmann SM: Comparison of Opa Locka Tower with other ATC facilities by means of a biochemical stress index. ADA008378

74-12   Smith RC: A realistic view of the people in air traffic control. ADA006789

1975

75-1   Jones KN, Steen JA, Collins WE: Predictive validities of several clinical color vision tests for aviation signal light gun performance. ADA006792

75-2   Snow CC, Reynolds HM, Allgood MA: Anthropometry of airline stewardesses. ADA012965

75-3   Mathews JJ, Cobb BB Jr, Collins WE: Attitudes on en route air traffic control training and work: A comparison of recruits initially trained at the FAA Academy and recruits initially trained at assigned centers. ADA013343

75-4   Collins WE, Lennon A0, Grimm EJ: The use of vestibular tests in civil aviation medical examinations: Survey of practices and proposals by aviation medical examiners. ADA015087

75-5   Ryan LC, Gerathewohl SJ, Mohler SR, Booze CF Jr: To see or not to see: Visual acuity of pilots involved in midair collisions. ADA016277

75-6   Lewis MF, Ferraro DP, Mertens HW, Steen JA: Interaction between marihuana and altitude on a complex behavioral task in baboons. ADA020680/5GI

75-7   Melton CE Jr, Smith RC, McKenzie JM, Saldivar JT, Hoffmann SM, Fowler PR: Stress in air traffic controllers: Comparison of two air route traffic control centers on different shift rotation patterns. ADA020679/7GI

75-8   Thackray RI, Bailey JP, Touchstone RM: Physiological, subjective, and performance correlates of reported boredom and monotony while performing a simulated radar control task. ADA025426/8GI

75-9   Smith RC, Rana B, Taylor DK: An evaluation of the effectiveness of the FAA Management Training School. ADA025254/4GI

75-10   Higgins EA, Chiles WD, McKenzie JM, Iampietro PF, Winget CM, Funkhouser GE, Burr MJ, Vaughan JA, Jennings AE: The effects of a 12-hour shift in the wake-sleep cycle on the physiological and biochemical responses and on multiple-task performance. ADA021518/GGI

75-11   Tobias JV: Earplug ratings based on the protector-attenuation rating (P-AR). ADA024756/9GI

75-12   Hasbrook AH, Rasmussen PG, Willis DM: Pilot performance and heart rate during in-flight use of a compact instrument display. ADA021519/4GI

75-13   Reynolds HM, Allgood MA: Functional strength of commercial-airline stewardesses. ADA021836/2GI

75-14   Higgins EA, Chiles WD, McKenzie JM, Iampietro PF, Vaughan JA, Funkhouser GE, Burr MJ, Jennings AE, West G: The effects of dextroamphetamine on physiological responses and complex performance during sleep loss. ADA021520/2GI

1976

76-1   Jennings AE, Chiles WD: An investigation of time-sharing ability as a factor in complex performance. ADA031881/GGA

76-2   Smith RC, Melton CE: Effects of ground trainer use on the psychological and physiological states of students in private pilot training. ADA024704/9GI

76-3   Tobias JV: Massed versus distributed practice in learned improvement of speech intelligibility. ADA024705/GGI

76-4   Constant GN, Grimm EJ, Goulden DR, Murcko LE: Aviation medicine translations: Annotated bibliography of recently translated material. IX. ADA031492/2GA

76-5   Vaughan JA, Welsh KW: Visual evaluation of smoke-protective devices. ADA031493/0GI

76-6   Cobb BB Jr, Young CL, Rizzuti BL: Education as a factor in the selection of air traffic controller trainees. ADA031880/8GI

76-7   Dille JR, Booze CF Jr: Accident experience of civilian pilots with static physical defects. ADA029431/4GI

76-8   Reighard HL: Aviation medicine. ADA032558/9GI

Part I: Chronological Index

76-9 Young JW, Reynolds HM, McConville JT, Snyder RG, Chandler RF: Development and evaluation of masterbody forms for 3- and 6-year-old-child dummies. ADA037547/7GI

76-10 Dark SJ: Characteristics of medically disqualified airman applicants in calendar years 1973 and 1974. ADA032603/3GI

76-11 Higgins EA, Chiles WD, McKenzie JM, Funkhouser GE, Burr MJ, Jennings AE, Vaughan JA: Physiological, biochemical, and multiple-task-performance responses to different alterations of the wake-sleep cycle. ADA033889/7GI

76-12 Collins WE: Some effects of sleep deprivation on tracking performance in static and dynamic environments. ADA033331/0GI

76-13 Melton CE Jr, Smith RC, McKenzie JM, Hoffmann SM, Saldivar JT: Stress in air traffic controllers: Effects of ARTS-III. ADA034752/GGI

76-14 Lentz JM, Collins WE: Three studies of motion sickness susceptibility. ADA036284/8GI

76-15 McKenzie JM: The aeromedical significance of sickle-cell trait. ADA038466/9GI

1977

77-1 Murcko LE, Dille JR: Index to FAA Office of Aviation Medicine Reports: 1961 through 1976. ADA037234/2GI

77-2 Welsh KW, Vaughan JA, Rasmussen PG: Survey of cockpit visual problems of senior pilots. ADA037587/3GI

77-3 Lategola MT, Flux M, Lyne PJ: Spirometric assessment of potential respiratory impairment in general aviation airmen. ADA038296/0

77-4 Valdez CD: Ten-year survey of altitude chamber reactions using the FAA training chamber flight profiles. ADA03723/9GI

77-5 Saldivar JT, Hoffmann SM, Melton CE: Sleep in air traffic controllers. ADA038297/8GI

77-6 Gerathewohl SJ: Psychophysiological effects of aging: Developing a functional age index for pilots: I. A survey of the pertinent literature. ADA04032/0GI

77-7 Welsh KW, Rasmussen PG, Vaughan JA: Intermediate visual acuity of presbyopic individuals with and without distance and bifocal lens corrections. ADA038538/5GI

77-8 Hanneman GD, Higgins EA, Price GT, Funkhouser GE, Grape PM, Snyder L: A study of effects of hyperthermia on large, short-haired male dogs: A simulated air transport environmental stress. ADA040432/7GI

77-9 Crane CR, Sanders DC, Endecott BR, Abbott JK, Smith PW: Inhalation toxicology: I. Design of a small-animal test system. II. Determination of the relative toxic hazards of 75 aircraft cabin materials. ADA043646/9GI

77-10 Booze CF Jr: An epidemiologic investigation of occupation, age, and exposure in general aviation accidents. ADA040978/9GI

77-11 Blethrow JG, Garner JD, Lowrey DL, Busby DE, Chandler RF: Emergency escape of handicapped air travelers. ADA043269/0GI

77-12 Mertens HW: Perceived orientation of a runway model in nonpilots during simulated night approaches to landing. ADA044553/GGI

77-13 Welsh KW, Rasmussen PG, Vaughan JA: Readability of alphanumeric characters having various contrast levels as a function of age and illumination mode. ADA044554/4GI

77-14 Welsh KW, Rasmussen PG, Vaughan JA: Refractive error characteristics of early and advanced presbyopic individuals. ADA044555/1GI

77-15 Chiles WD: Objective methods for developing indices of pilot workload. ADA044556/9GI

77-16 Lategola MT, Flux M, Lyne PJ: Altitude tolerance of general aviation pilots with normal or partially impaired spirometric function. ADA044557/7GI

77-17 Higgins EA, Chiles WD, McKenzie JM, Davis AW Jr, Funkhouser GE, Jennings AE, Mullen SR, Fowler PR: Effects of lithium carbonate on performance and biomedical functions. ADA044824/1GI

77-18 Thackray RI, Bailey JP, Touchstone RM: The effect of increased monitoring load on vigilance performance using a simulated radar display. ADA044558/5GI

77-19 Smith PW, Robinson CP, Zelenski JD, Endecott BR: The role of monamine oxidase inhibition in the acute toxicity of chlordimeform. ADA045507/1GI

77-20 Dille JR, Booze CF: The 1975 accident experience of civilian pilots with static physical defects. ADA045429/8GI

77-21 Smith RC, Hutto GL: Job attitudes of airway facilities personnel. ADA04641/3GI

77-22 Revzin AM: Functional localization in the nucleus rotundus. ADA047717/4GI

77-23 Melton CE, Smith RC, McKenzie JM, Wicks SM, Saldivar JT: Stress in air traffic personnel: Low-density towers and flight service stations. ADA046826/4GI

77-24 Collins WE, Hasbrook AH, Lennon A0, Gay DJ: Disorientation training in FAA-certificated flight and ground schools: a survey. ADA047718/2GI

77-25 Dailey JT, Pickrel EW: Development of new selection tests for air traffic controllers. ADA049049/0GI

1978

78-1 McFadden EB, (Ed.): Flotation and survival equipment studies. ADA051869/GGI

78-2 Revzin AM: Effects of ethanol on visual unit activity in the thalamus. ADA05092/4GI

78-3 Pollard DW, Garner JD, Blethrow JG, Lowrey DL: Passenger flow rates between compartments: Straight-segmented stairways, spiral stairways, and passageways with restricted vision and changes of attitude. ADA05148/1GI

78-4 deSteiguer D, Pinski MS, Bannister JR, McFadden EB: Aircrew and passenger protective breathing equipment studies. ADA05100/4GI

78-5 Higgins EA, Lategola MT, Melton CE: Three reports relevant to stress in aviation personnel. ADA051690/GGI

78-6 Chandler RF, Trout EM: Evaluation of seating and restraint systems and anthropomorphic dummies conducted during fiscal year 1976. ADA051691/4GI

78-7 Lewis MA: Use of the occupational knowledge test to assign extra credit in selection of air traffic controllers. ADA05367/5GI

78-8 Friedberg W, Neas BR, Faulkner DN, Hanneman GD, Darden EB Jr: Radiobiological aspects of high altitude flight: Relative biological effectiveness of fast neutrons in suppressing immune capacity to an infective agent. ADA05320/4GI

78-9 McFadden EB: Human respiratory considerations for civil transport aircraft system. ADA053223/4GI

78-10 Boone J0: The relationship of predevelopmental "150" training with noncompetitively selected air traffic control trainees to FAA Academy success. ADA055009/5GI

78-11 Thackray RI, Touchstone RM, Bailey JP: A comparison of the vigilance performance of men and women using a simulated radar task. ADA053674/8GI

78-12 Chandler RF, Trout EM: Child restraint systems for civil aircraft. ADA053565/8GI

78-13 Kirkham WR, Collins WE, Grape PM, Simpson JM, Wallace TF: Spatial disorientation in general aviation accidents. ADA053230/9GI

78-14 Young JW, Pinski MS: Three-dimensional anthropometry of the adult face. ADA054938/GGI

78-15 Mertens HW: Comparison of the visual perception of a runway model in pilots and nonpilots during simulated night landing approaches. ADA054450/2GI

78-16 Gerathewohl SJ: Psychophysiological effects of aging: Developing a functional age index for pilots: II. Taxonomy of psychological factors. ADA054356/1GI

78-17 Rasmussen PG, Welsh KW, Vaughan JA: Comparative readability of enroute low altitude charts with and without terrain depiction. ADA054796/8GI

78-18 Melton CE, McKenzie JM, Saldivar JT, Wicks SM: Experimental attempts to evoke a differential response to different stressors. ADA054795/0GI

78-19 Higgins EA, Chiles WD, McKenzie JM, Jennings AE, Funkhouser GE, Mullen SR: The effects of altitude and two decongestant-antihistamine preparations on physiological functions and performance. ADA054793/5GI

78-20 Lategola MT, Davis AW Jr, Lyne PJ, Burr MJ: Cardiorespiratory assessment of decongestant-antihistamine effects on altitude, +Gz, and fatigue tolerances. ADA055089/7GI

78-21 Booze CF: The morbidity experience of air traffic control personnel, 1967-1977. ADA056053/26I

78-22 Welsh KW, Vaughan JA, Rasmussen PG: Aeromedical implications of the X-Chrom lens for improving color vision deficiencies. ADA054794/3GI

78-23 Garner JD, Chandler RF, Cook EA: GPSS computer simulation of aircraft passenger emergency evacuations. ADA056098/7GI

Part I: Chronological Index

78-24 Chandler RF, Trout EM: Evaluation of seating and restraint systems and anthropomorphic dummies conducted during fiscal year 1977. ADA056905/3GI

78-25 Dark SJ, Davis AW Jr: Characteristics of medically disqualified airman applicants in calendar years 1975 and 1976. ADA058158/7GI

78-26 Robinson CP, Beiergrohslein D, Smith PW, Crane CR: Reactions of methamidophos with mammalian cholinesterases. ADA058683/4GI

78-27 Gerathewohl SJ: Psychophysiological effects of aging: Developing a functional age index for pilots: III. Measurement of pilot performance. ADA062501/2GA

78-28 Welsh KW, Rasmussen PG, Vaughan JA: Visual performance assessment through clear and sunscreen-treated windows. ADA059750/0GA

78-29 Welsh KW, Vaughan JA, Rasmussen PG: Conspicuity assessment of selected propeller and tail rotor paint schemes. ADA061875/1GA

78-30 McKenzie JM: Assessment of factors possibly contributing to the susceptibility of sickle trait erythrocytes to mild hypoxia. ADA056200/9GI

78-31 Lacefield DJ, Roberts PA, Blossom CW: Agricultural aviation versus other general aviation: Toxicological findings in fatal accidents. ADA060110/4GA

78-32 Smith RC: As evaluation of four MTS recurrent training courses. ADA061519/5GA

78-33 Chiles WD, Jennings AE: Time-sharing ability in complex performance: An expanded replication. ADA061879/3GA

78-34 Chiles WD, Jennings AE, Alluisi EA: The measurement and scaling of workload in complex performance. ADA061725/8GA

78-35 Reighard HL, Dailey JT: Task force deterrence of air piracy-final report. ADA076457/1

78-36 Boone J0, Lewis MA: The development of the ATC selection battery: A new procedure to make maximum use of available information when correcting correlations for restriction in range due to selection. ADA066131/2GA

78-37 Jennings AE: A method to evaluate performance reliability of individual subjects in laboratory research applied to work settings. ADA063731/4GA

78-38 Eighth Bethesda Conference of the American College of Cardiology Washington D.C. April 25-26 1975: Cardiovascular problems associated with aviation safety. ADA066184/3GA

78-39 Rose RM, Jenkins CD, Hurst MW: Air traffic controller health change study. Boston University School of Medicine. ADA063709/0GA

78-40 Melton CE, McKenzie JM, Wicks SM, Saldivar JT: Stress in air traffic controllers: A restudy of 32 controllers 5 to 9 years later. ADA065767/6GA

78-41 Vaughan JA, Welsh KW, Rasmussen PG: The optical properties of smoke-protective devices. ADA064678/6GA

1979

79-1 Index to FAA Office of Aviation Medicine Reports: 1961 through 1978. ADA067983/7GA

79-2 Snow CC, Hartman S, Giles E, Young FA: Sex and race determination of crania by calipers and computer: A test of the Giles and Elliot discriminant functions in 52 forensic cases. ADA065448/36A

79-3 Lewis MA: A comparison of three models for determining test fairness. ADA066586/9GA

79-4 Lewis MF, Mertens HW: Pilot performance during simulated approaches and landings made with various computer-generated visual glidepath indicators. ADA066220/5GA

79-5 Tobias JV, Kidd GD Jr: Accoustic signals for emergency evacuation. ADA066113/2.A

79-6 Pollard DW: Injuries in air transport emergency evacuations. ADA069372/1GA

79-7 Collins WE, Chiles WD: Laboratory performance during acute intoxication and hangover. ADA069373/9GA

79-8 Lategola MT, Trent CC: A lower body negative pressure box for +Gz simulation in the upright seated position. ADA069326/7GA

79-9 Schroeder DJ, Collins WE: Effects of congener and noncongener alcoholic beverages on a clinical ataxia battery. ADA069375/4GA

79-10   Higgins EA, McKenzie JM, Funkhouser GE, Mullen SR: Effects of propranolol on time of useful function (TUF) in rats. ADA068535/4GA

79-11   Smith RC: A comparison of the job attitudes and interest patterns of air traffic and airway facility personnel. ADA067826/8GA

79-12   Thackray RI, Touchstone RM: Visual search performance during simulated radar observation with and without a sweepline. ADA068020/7GA

79-13   McFadden EB, (Ed.): Oxygen equipment and rapid decompression studies. ADA070285/2GA

79-14   Boone J0, Lewis MA: The selection of air traffic control specialists: Two studies demonstrating methods to insure an accurate validity coefficient for selection devices. ADA068581/8GA

79-15   Revzin AM: Development of electrophysiological indices of neurological toxicity for organophosphate pesticides and depressant drugs. ADA070299/3GA

79-16   Tobias JV: Interstimulus interval as it affects temporary threshold shift in serial presentations of loud tones. ADA072006/0GA

79-17   Chandler RF, Trout EM: Evaluation of seating and restraint systems conducted during fiscal year 1978. ADA074881/4

79-18   Pickrel EW: Performance standards for pass-fail determinations in the national air traffic flight service station training program. ADA081066/3

79-19   Dille JR, Booze CF: The 1976 accident experience of civilian pilots with static physical defects. ADA07718919

79-20   Higgins EA, Lategola MT, McKenzie JM, Melton CE, Vaughan JA: Effects of ozone on exercising and sedentary adult men and women representative of the flight attendant population. ADA080045/8

79-21   Boone JO: Toward the development of a new selection battery for air traffic control specialists. ADA080065/6

79-22   Rasmussen PG, Garner JD, Blethrow JG, Lowrey DL: Readability of self-illuminated signs in a smoke-obscured environment. ADA081260/2

79-23   Pollard DW, Anderson JA, Melton RJ: A description of the Civil Aeromedical Institute airline cabin safety data bank: 1970-1976. ADA081155/4

79-24   Thackray RI, Touchstone RM: Effects of noise exposure on performance of a simulated radar task. ADA081065/5

79-25   Mertens HW: Runway image as a cue for judgment of approach angle. ADA080929/3

79-26   Collins WE: Performance effects of alcohol intoxication and hangover at ground level and at simulated altitude. ADA079439/6

1980

80-1   Thackray RI: Boredom and monotony as a consequence of automation: A consideration of the evidence relating boredom and monotony to stress. ADA085069/3

80-2   Friedberg W, Neas BR (Eds.): Cosmic radiation exposure during air travel. ADA084801/0

80-3   Kirkham WR, Simpson JM, Wallace TF, Grape PM: Aircraft crashworthiness studies: Findings in accidents involving an aerial application aircraft. ADA084619/6

80-4   Ryan LC, Mohler SR: The current role of alcohol as a factor in civil aircraft accidents. ADA086261/5

80-5   Boone JO, Steen JA, VanBuskirk LK: System performance, error rates, and training time for recent FAA Academy nonradar graduates, community persons, and handicapped persons on the radar training facility pilot position. ADA087661/5

80-6   Kirkham WR: Medical and toxicological factors in aircraft accidents. ADA087690/4

80-7   Collins WE, Boone JO, VanDeventer AD (Eds.): The selection of air traffic control specialists: I. History and review of contributions by the Civil Aeromedical Institute. ADA087655/7

80-8   Booze CF, Pidkowicz JK, Davis AW, Bolding FA: Postmortem coronary atherosclerosis findings in general aviation accident pilot fatalities: 1975-1977. ADA089428/7

80-9   Higgins EA, Lategola MT, Melton CE, Vaughan JA: Effects of ozone (0.30 parts per million, ~600 ug/m3) on sedentary men representative of airline passengers and cockpit crewmembers. ADA092268/2

80-10   McKenzie JM, Higgins EA, Funkhouser GE, Moses R, Fowler PR, Wicks SM: Changes in the oxygen-hemoglobin dissociation curve and time of useful function at hypobaric pressures in rats after chronic oral administration of propranolol. ADA089139/0

Part I: Chronological Index

80-11 Dille JR, Linder MK: The effects of tobacco on aviation safety. ADA091510/8

80-12 Chandler RF, Garner JD, Lowrey DL, Blethrow JG, Anderson JA: Considerations relative to the use of canes by blind travelers in air carrier aircraft cabins. ADA092528/9

80-13 Rasmussen PG, Chesterfield BP, Lowrey DL: Readability of self-illuminated signs obscured by black fuel-fire smoke. ADA092529/7

80-14 Smith RC: Stress, anxiety, and the air traffic control specialist: Some conclusions from a decade of research. ADA093266/5

80-15 Boone JO, Van Buskirk L, Steen JA: The Federal Aviation Administration's radar training facility and employee selection and training. ADA093027/1

80-16 Melton CE: Effects of long-term exposure to low levels of ozone: A review. ADA094426/4

80-17 Thackray RI, Touchstone RM: An exploratory investigation of various assessment instruments as correlates of complex visual monitoring performance. ADA097276/0

80-18 deSteiguer D, Saldivar JT: Evaluation of the protective efficiency of a new oxygen mask for aircraft passenger use to 40,000 feet. ADA097046/7

80-19 Dark SJ: Characteristics of medically disqualified airman applicants in calendar years 1977 and 1978. ADA098766/9

80-20 McKenzie JM: Vocational options for those with sickle cell trait: Questions about hypoxemia and the industrial environment. ADA098706/5

1981

81-1 Dille JR, Haraway A: Index to FAA Office of Aviation Medicine Reports: 1961 through 1980. ADA106227/2

81-2 Lategola MT, Lyne PJ, Burr MJ: Cardiorespiratory assessment of 24-hour crash-diet effects on altitude, +Gz, and fatigue tolerances. ADA106379/1

81-3 Federal Aviation Administration Contract DOT-FA-77WA-4076: Neurological and neurosurgical conditions associated with aviation safety. ADA098697/6

81-4 Simpson LP, Goulden DR: Aviation medicine translations: Annotated bibliography of recently translated material. X. ADA098916/0

81-5 Hutto GL, Smith RC, Thackray RI: Methodology in the assessment of stress among air traffic control specialists (ATCS): Normative adult data for the State-Trait Anxiety Inventory from non-ATCS populations. ADA103192/1

81-6 Mertens HW, Lewis MF: Effect of different runway size on pilot performance during simulated night landing approaches. ADA103190/5

81-7 Chesterfield BP, Rasmussen PG, Dillon RD: Emergency cabin lighting installations: An analysis of ceiling- vs. lower-cab-inmounted lighting during evacuation trials. ADA103191/3

81-8 Higgins EA, Mertens HM, McKenzie JW, Funkhouser GE: Physiological, biochemical, and performance responses to a 24-hour crash diet. ADA103143/4

81-9 Booze CF Jr: Prevalence of selected pathology among currently certified active airman. ADA103397/6

81-10 Kirkham WR: Improving the crashworthiness of general aviation aircraft by crash injury investigations. ADA103316/6

81-11 Hanneman GD: Factors related to the welfare of animals during transport by commercial aircraft. ADA106226/4

81-12 Thackray RI, Touchstone RM: Age-related differences in complex monitoring performance. ADA106225/6

81-13 Melton CE, McKenzie JM, Wicks SM, Saldivar JT: Fatigue in flight inspection field office (FIFO) flight crews. ADA106791/7

81-14 Dille JR, Booze CF Jr: The prevalence of visual deficiencies among 1979 general aviation accident airmen. ADA106489/8

81-15 Collins WE, Mastrullo AR, Kirkham WR, Taylor DK, Grape PM: An analysis of civil aviation propeller-to-person accidents: 1965-1979. ADA105365/1

81-16 Collins WE, Schroeder DJ, Elam GW: A comparison of some effects of three antimotion sickness drugs on nystagmic responses to angular accelerations and to optokinetic stimuli. ADA107947/4

1982

82-1 Thackray RI, Touchstone RM: Performance of air traffic control specialists (ATCS's) on a laboratory radar monitoring task: An exploratory study of complacency and a comparison of ATCS and non-ATCS performance ADA118239/3

82-2 Boone J0: A generic model for evaluation of the Federal Aviation Administration air traffic control specialist training programs. ADA106379/1

82-3 Lategola MT, Lyne PJ, Burr MJ: Alcohol-induced physiological displacements and their effects on flight-related functions. ADA115473/1

82-4 Lategola MT, Lyne PJ, Burr MJ: Effects of prior physical exertion on tolerance to hypoxia, orthostatic stress, and physical fatigue. ADA114741/2

82-5 Lategola MT, Flux M: Evaluation of cardiopulmonary factors critical to successful emergency perinatal air transport. ADA114743/8

82-6 Mertens HW, Lewis MF: Effects of approach lighting and variation in visible runway length on perception of approach angle in simulated night landings. ADA114742/0

82-7 Kirkham WR, Wicks SM, Lowrey DL: Crashworthiness studies: Cabin, seat, restraint, and injury findings in selected general aviation accidents. ADA114878/2

82-8 Pollard DW, Folk ED, Chandler RF: Flight attendant injuries: 1971-1976. ADA114909/5

82-9 Reynolds HM, Snow CC, Young JW: Spatial geometry of the human pelvis. ADA118238/5

82-10 Higgins EA, Mertens HW, McKenzie JM, Funkhouser GE, White MA, Milburn NJ: The effects of physical fatigue and altitude on physiological, biochemical, and performance responses. ADA122796/6

82-11 Rock DB, Dailey JT, Ozur H, Boone JO, Pickrel EW: Selection of applicants for the air traffic controller occupation. ADA122795/8

82-12 Friedberg W, Faulkner DN, Snyder L: Transport index limits for shipments of radioactive material in passenger-carrying aircraft. ADA122794/1

82-13 Kirkham WR, Wicks SM, Lowrey DL: G incapacitation in aerobatic pilots: A flight hazard. ADA123757/7

82-14 Norwood G, Jordan JL: Regulatory aviation medicine: Its philosophies and limitations. ADA124043/1

82-15 Lacefield DJ, Roberts PA, Grape PM: Carbon monoxide in-flight incapacitation: An occasional toxic problem in aviation. ADA123849/2

82-16 Thackray RI, Touchstone RM: Performance of 40- to 50-year- old subjects on a radar monitoring task: The effects of wearing bifocal glasses and interpolated rest periods on target detection time. ADA123843/5

82-17 Melton CE: Physiological stress in air traffic controllers: A review. ADA123853/4

82-18 Boone JO: Functional aging in pilots: An examination of a mathematical model based on medical data on general aviation pilots. ADA123756/9

82-19 Schroeder DJ, Collins WE, Elam GW: Effects of some motion sickness suppressants on tracking performance during angular accelerations. ADA123839/3

1983

83-1 Dille JR, Haraway A: Index to FAA Office of Aviation Medicine Reports: 1961 through 1982. ADA127463/8

83-2 McKenzie JM, Higgins EA, Fowler PR, Funkhouser GE, White MA, Moser E: Sensitivity of some tests for alcohol abuse: Findings in nonalcoholics recovering from intoxication. ADA126138/7

83-3 Coltman JW: Design and test criteria for increased energy-absorbing seat effectiveness. ADA1280125/5

83-4 Mertens HW, McKenzie JM, Higgins EA: Some effects of smoking withdrawal on complex performance and physiological responses. ADA126551/1

83-5 Dark SJ: Characteristics of medically disqualified airline pilots. ADA127429/9

83-6 VanDeventer AD, Taylor DK, Collins WE, Boone JO: Three studies of biographical factors associated with success in air traffic control specialist screening/training at the FAA Academy. ADA128784/6

83-7 Schroeder DJ, Deloney JR: Job attitudes toward the new maintenance concept of the Airway Facilities Service. ADA133282/4

83-8   Kirkham WR, Wicks SM, Lowrey DL: Crashworthiness: An illustrated commentary on occupant survival in general aviation accidents. ADA130198/5

83-9   Boone JO: Radar Training Facility initial validation. ADA133220/4

83-10 deSteiguer D, Saldivar JT: An analysis of potential breathing devices intended for use by aircraft passengers. ADA132648/7

83-11 Pickrel EW, Convey JJ: Color perception and ATC job performance. ADA132649/5

83-12 Crane CR, Sanders DC, Endecott BR, Abbott JK: Inhalation toxicology: III. Evaluation of thermal degradation products from aircraft and automobile engine oils, aircraft hydraulic fluid, and mineral oil. ADA133221/2

83-13 Thackray RI, Touchstone RM: Rate of initial recovery and subsequent radar monitoring performance following a simulated emergency involving startle. ADA133602/3

83-14 deSteiguer D, Saldivar JT, Higgins EA, Funkhouser GE: The objective evaluation of aircrew protective breathing equipment: V. Mask/goggles combinations for female crewmembers. ADA134912

83-15 Mertens HW, Higgins EA, McKenzie JM: Age, altitude, and workload effects on complex performance. ADA133594/2

83-16 Young JW, Chandler RF, Snow CC, Robinette KM, Zehner GF, Lofberg MS: Anthropometric and mass distribution characteristics of the adult female. ADA135316

83-17 Schroeder DJ, Goulden DR: A bibliography of shift work research: 1950-1982. ADA135644

83-18 Dille JR, Booze CF, Jr: The 1980 and 1981 accident experience of civil airmen with selected visual pathology. ADA134898

1984

84-1   Pollard DW, Steen JA, Biron WJ, Cremer RL: Cabin safety subject index. ADA140409

84-2   Sells SB, Dailey JT, Pickrel EW: Selection of air traffic controllers. ADA147765

84-3   Booze CF Jr, Simcox LS: Blood pressure levels of active pilots compared with those of air traffic controllers. ADA146645

84-4   Lategola MT, Davis AW Jr, Gilcher RO, Lyne PJ, Burr MJ: Aviation-related cardiorespiratory effects of blood donation in female private pilots. ADA148045

84-5   Hanneman GD, Sershon JL: Tolerance endpoint for evaluating the effects of heat stress in dogs. ADA148104

84-6   VanDeventer AD, Collins WE, Manning CA, Taylor DK, Baxter NE: Studies of poststrike air traffic control specialist trainees: I. Age, biographic factors, and selection test performance related to Academy training success. ADA147892

84-7   Dille JR, Harris JL: Efforts to improve aviation medical examiner performance through continuing medical education and annual performance reports. ADA148078

84-8   Booze CF Jr: Health examination findings among active civil airmen. ADA148325

84-9   Dark SJ: Medically disqualified airline pilots. ADA149454

1985

85-1   Pollard DW, Steen JA, Penland T: Federal Aviation Regulations Part 135 cabin safety subject index. ADA156946

85-2   Melton CE: Physiological responses to unvarying (steady) and 2-2-1 shifts: Miami International Flight Service Station. ADA155751

85-3   Mertens HW, Collins WE: The effects of age, sleep deprivation, and altitude on complex performance. ADA156987

85-4   Crane CR, Sanders DC, Endecott BR, Abbott JK: Inhalation toxicology: IV. Times to incapacitation and death for rats exposed continuously to atmospheric hydrogen chloride gas. ADA157400

85-5   Collins WE, Mertens HW, Higgins EA: Some effects of alcohol and simulated altitude on complex performance scores and Breathalyzer readings. ADA158925

85-6   Booze CF Jr, Staggs CM: A comparison of postmortem coronary atherosclerosis findings in general aviation pilot fatalities. ADA159811

85-7   Convey JJ: Passing scores for the FAA ATCS color vision test. ADA160889

85-8   Lacefield DJ, Roberts PA, Grape PM: Drugs of abuse in aviation fatalities: 1. Marijuana. ADA161911

85-9   Dark SJ: Characteristics of medically disqualified airman applicants in calendar years 1982 and 1983. ADA162209

85-10 Higgins EA, Saldivar JT, Lyne PJ, Funkhouser GE: Evaluation of a passenger mask modified with a rebreather bag for protection from smoke and fumes. ADA162473

85-11 Rueschhoff BJ, Higgins EA, Burr MJ, Branson DM: Development and evaluation of a prototype life preserver. ADA163224

85-12 Russell JC, Davis AW: Alcohol rehabilitation of airline pilots. ADA163076

85-13 Thackray RI, Touchstone RM: The effect of visual taskload on critical flicker frequency (CFF) change during performance of a complex monitoring task. ADA163673

1986

86-1 Sanders DC, Crane CR, Endecott BR: Inhalation toxicology: V. Evaluation of relative toxicity to rats of thermal decomposition products from two aircraft seat fire-blocking materials. ADA165034

86-2 Melton CE, Bartanowicz RS: Biological rhythms and rotating shift work: Some considerations for air traffic controllers and managers. ADA168742

86-3 Crane CR, Sanders DC, Endecott BR, Abbott JK: Inhalation toxicology: VI. Evaluation of the relative toxicity of thermal decomposition products from nine aircraft panel materials, ADA168250

86-4 Thackray RI, Touchstone RM: Complex monitoring performance and the coronary-prone Type A behavior pattern. ADA168240

86-5 Crane CR, Sanders DC, Endecott BR, Abbott JK: Inhalation toxicology: VII. Times to incapacitation and death for rats exposed continuously to atmospheric acrolein vapor.

86-6 Convey JJ: The Flight Service Station Training Program: 1981-1985. ADA171485

86-7 Dark SJ: Medically disqualified airline pilots. ADA173244

86-8 Crane CR, Sanders DC: Inhalation toxicology: VIII. Establishing heat tolerance limits for rats and mice subjected to acute exposures at elevated air temperatures. ADA173031

86-9 Collins WE: Effects of sleep loss on vestibular responses during simple and complex vestibular stimulation. ADA173292

1987

87-1 Dille JR, Grimm MH: Index to FAA Office of Aviation Medicine Reports: 1961 through 1986. ADA180281

87-2 Higgins EA, Saldivar JT, Lyne PJ, Funkhouser GE: A study of passenger workload as related to protective breathing requirements. ADA181089

87-3 Hanneman GD, Sershon JL: Tolerance by unacclimated Beagle dogs to freezing and subfreezing temperatures. ADA181304

87-4 Schroeder DJ, Collins WE, Dollar CS: 1986 survey of aviation business operators: Their views of FAA airworthiness inspectors. ADA181369

87-5 Higgins EA: Summary report of the history and events pertinent to the Civil Aeromedical Institute's evaluation of providing smoke/fume protective breathing equipment for airline passenger use. ADA184499

87-6 Diehl AE, Lester LF: Private pilot judgment training in flight school settings. ADA188408

87-7 Booze CF Jr: Sudden in-flight incapacitation in general aviation. ADA187044

87-8 Hanneman GD, Sershon JL: A temperature/humidity tolerance index for transporting Beagle dogs in hot weather. ADA190948

1988

88-1 Thackray RI, Touchstone RM: An evaluation of the effects of high visual taskload on the separate behaviors involved in complex monitoring performance. ADA190641

88-2 Collins WE, Mertens HW: Age, alcohol, and simulated altitude: Effects on performance and breathalyzer scores. ADA190642

88-3 Manning CA, Kegg PS, Collins WE: Studies of poststrike air traffic control specialist trainees: II. Selection and Screening. ADA199177

Part I: Chronological Index

88-4 Thackray RI: Performance recovery following startle: a laboratory approach to the study of behavioral response to sudden aircraft emergencies. ADA199827

88-5 Clough DL: Airway science curriculum demonstration project: Summary of initial evaluation findings. ADA201995

1989

89-1 Thackray RI, Touchstone RM: A comparison of detection efficiency on an air traffic control monitoring task with and without computer aiding. ADA206422

89-2 Booze CF Jr: Prevalence of disease among active civil airmen. ADA206050

89-3 Colangelo EJ, Russell JC: Injuries to seat occupants of light airplanes. ADA207579

89-4 Crane CR, Sanders DC, Endecott, BR: Inhalation toxicology: IX. Times-to-incapacitation for rats exposed to carbon monoxide alone, to hydrogen cyanide alone, to mixtures of carbon monoxide and hydrogen cyanide. ADA208195

89-5 Higgins EA, Vant JHB: Operation Workload - A study of passenger energy expenditure during an emergency evacuation. ADA209234

89-6 Manning CA, Della Rocco PS, Bryant KD: Prediction of success in FAA air traffic control field training as a function of selection and screening test performance. ADA209327

89-7 Collins WE, Schroeder DJ, Nye LG: Relationships of anxiety scores to Academy and field training performance of air traffic control specialists. ADA209326

89-8 Higgins EA, McLean GA, Lyne PJ, Funkhouser GE, Young JW: Performance evaluation of the Puritan-Bennett crewmember portable protective breathing device as prescribed by portions of FAA Action Notice A-8150.2. ADA210882

89-9 Shepherd WT, Parker JF Jr: Human factors issues in aircraft maintenance and inspection. ADA215 724

89-10 Schlegel TT, Higgins EA, McLean GA, Lyne PJ, England HM, Atocknie PA: Comparison of protective breathing equipment performance at ground level and 8,000 feet altitude using parameters prescribed by portions of FAA Action Notice A-8150.2. ADA212852

89-11 Higgins EA, McLean GA, Lyne PJ, Funkhouser GE, Young JW: Evaluation of the Scott Aviation portable protective breathing device for contaminant leakage as prescribed by FAA Action Notice A-8150.2. ADA216799

89-12 McLean GA, Higgins EA, Lyne PJ: The effects of wearing passenger protective breathing equipment on evacuation times through type III and type IV emergency aircraft exits in clear air and smoke. ADA216798

89-13 Melton CE: Airliner cabin ozone: an updated review. ADA233156.

89-14 Rasmussen PB, Chittum CG: The influence of adjacent seating configurations on egress through a type III emergency exit. ADA218393

1990

90-1 Collins WE, Wayda ME, Baxter NE: Index of FAA Office of Aviation Medicine Reports: 1961 through 1989. AD-221414

90-2 Myers JG: Management assessment: implications for development and training. ADA219178

90-3 Thackray RI, Touchstone RM: Effects of monitoring under high and low taskload on detection of flashing and colored radar targets. ADA220313

90-4 Collins WE, Nye LG, Manning CA: Studies of poststrike air traffic control specialist trainees: III. Changes in demographic characteristics of Academy entrants and biodemographic predictors of success in air traffic controller selection and Academy screening. ADA223480

90-5 Downey LE, Dark SJ: Medically disqualified airline pilots in calendar years 1987 and 1988. ADA224512

90-6 Manning CA, Schroeder DJ: Pilot views of Montgomery County, Texas automated FSS services. ADA227484

90-7 Hudson LS, Booze CF Jr Davis AW: Right bundle branch block as a risk factor for subsequent cardiac events. ADA226596

90-8 Schroeder DJ, Dollar CS, Nye LG: Correlates of two experimental tests with performance in the FAA Academy air traffic control nonradar screen program. ADA226419

90-9 Mertens HW: Evaluation of functional color vision requirements and current color vision screening tests for air traffic control specialists. ADA227436

90-10   Nakagawara VB: The use of contact lenses in the civil airman population. ADA227450

90-11   Gowdy V: Development of a crashworthy seat for commuter aircraft. ADA227486

90-12   Valdez CD: The FAA altitude chamber training flight profile: A survey of altitude reactions - 1965-1989. ADA230057

90-13   Della Rocco PS, Manning CA: Selection of air traffic controllers for automated systems: applications from current research. ADA230058

90-14   Parker JF Jr, Shepherd WT, Co-editors: Second Federal Aviation Administration meeting on human factors issues in aircraft maintenance and inspection: Information exchange and communications. ADA230270

90-15   Crane CR, Sanders DC, Endecott BR: Inhalation toxicology: X. Times to incapacitation for rats exposed continuously to carbon monoxide, acrolein, to carbon monoxide-acrolein mixtures. ADA230639

90-16   Sanders DC, Endecott BR: Inhalation toxicology: XI. The effect of elevated temperature on carbon monoxide toxicity. ADA231185

90-4   Collins WE, Nye LG, Manning CA: Studies of poststrike air traffic control specialist trainees: III. Changes in demographic characteristics of Academy entrants and biodemographic predictors of success in air traffic controller selection and Academy screening. ADA223480

90-5   Downey LE, Dark SJ: Medically disqualified airline pilots in calendar years 1987 and 1988. ADA224512

90-6   Manning CA, Schroeder DJ: Pilot views of Montgomery County, Texas automated FSS services. ADA227484

90-7   Hudson LS, Booze CF Jr Davis AW: Right bundle branch block as a risk factor for subsequent cardiac events. ADA226596

90-8   Schroeder DJ, Dollar CS, Nye LG: Correlates of two experimental tests with performance in the FAA Academy air traffic control nonradar screen program. ADA226419

90-9   Mertens HW: Evaluation of functional color vision requirements and current color vision screening tests for air traffic control specialists. ADA227436

90-10   Nakagawara VB: The use of contact lenses in the civil airman population. ADA227450

90-11   Gowdy V: Development of a crashworthy seat for commuter aircraft. ADA227486

90-12   Valdez CD: The FAA altitude chamber training flight profile: A survey of altitude reactions — 1965-1989. ADA230057

90-13   Della Rocco PS, Manning CA: Selection of air traffic controllers for automated systems: applications from current research. ADA230058

90-14   Parker JF Jr, Shepherd WT, Co-editors: Second Federal Aviation Administration meeting on human factors issues in aircraft maintenance and inspection: Information exchange and communications. ADA230270

90-15   Crane CR, Sanders DC, Endecott BR: Inhalation toxicology: X. Times to incapacitation for rats exposed continuously to carbon monoxide, acrolein, to carbon monoxide-acrolein mixtures. ADA230639

90-16   Sanders DC, Endecott BR: Inhalation toxicology: XI. The effect of elevated temperature on carbon monoxide toxicity. ADA231185

1991

91-1   Nakagawara VB: The effect of simulated altitude on the visual fields of glaucoma patients and the elderly. ADA233167

91-2   Hordinsky JR, George, MH: Utilization of emergency medical kits by air carriers. ADA234784

91-3   Hordinsky JR, George MH: Response capability during civil air carrier inflight medical emergencies. ADA235526

91-4   Broach D: Flight service specialist initial qualifications course: Content validation of FAA Academy course 50232. ADA237126

91-5   Myers JG, Stutzman TM: Job task-competency linkages for FAA first-level supervisors. ADA236695

91-6   Funkhouser GE, Fairlie GW: Donning times and flotation characteristics of infant life preservers: Four representative types. ADA237120

91-7   Turner JW, Huntley MS Jr: The use and design of flightcrew checklists and manuals. ADA237206

91-8   Nye LG, Collins WE: Some personality characteristics of air traffic control specialist trainees: Interactions of personality and aptitude test scores with FAA Academy success and career expectations. ADA238027

Part I: Chronological Index

91-9 Wing H, Manning CA: Selection of air traffic controllers: Complexity, requirements, and public interest. ADA238267

91-10 Witt LA, Myers JG: Two studies on participation in decision-making and equity among FAA personnel. ADA239907

91-11 Witt LA, Broach D: Exchange ideology as a moderator of the procedural justice-satisfaction relationship. ADA239908

91-12 McLean GA, Wilcox B.C, Canfield DV: Selection criteria for alcohol detection methods. ADA240441

91-13 Turner JW, Huntley MS Jr: Civilian training in high-altitude flight physiology. ADA241296

91-14 Nakagawara VB, Loochan FK, Wood KJ: The prevalence of aphakia in the civil airman population. ADA214032

91-15 Witt LA, Hellman CM: Cross-level inferences of job satisfaction in the prediction of intent to leave. ADA242779

91-16 Shepherd WB, Johnson WB, Druray CG, Taylor JC, Berninger D: Human factors in aviation maintenance. Phase 1: Progress report. ADA243844

91-17 Sanders DC, Endecott BS, Chaturvedi AK: Inhalation toxicology: XII. Comparison of toxicity rankings of six polymers in lethality and by incapacitation in rats. ADA244599

91-18 Broach D: Air traffic control specialists in the Airway Science Curriculum Demonstration Project 1984-1990: Third summative evaluation. ADA244128

1992

92-1 Collins WE, Wayda ME: Index of FAA Office of Aviation Medicine Reports: 1961 through 1991. ADA245509

92-2 Friedberg W, Snyder L, Faulkner DN: Radiation exposure of air carrier crewmembers II. ADA245508

92-3 Thackray RI: Human factors evaluation of the work environment of operators engaged in the inspection and repair of aging aircraft. ADA246445

92-4 May ND: Exposures from headset interference tones. ADA247175

92-5 Manning CA, Aul JC: Evaluation of an alternative method for hiring air traffic control specialists with prior military experience. ADA246587

92-6 Mertens HW, Thackray RI, Touchstone M: Effects of color vision deficiency on detection of color-highlighted targets in a simulated air traffic control display. ADA246586

92-7 Nye LG, Witt LA, Schroeder D: Confirmatory factor analysis of burnout dimensions: Correlations with job stressors and aspects of social support and job satisfaction ADA247699

92-8 Witt LA, Nye LG: Organizational goal congruence and job attitudes revisited. ADA247621

92-9 Witt LA, Nye LG: Gender, equity and job satisfaction. ADA246588

92-10 Nye LG, Witt LA: Dimensionality and construct validity of the Perceptions of Organizational Politics Scale (POPS). ADA247620

92-11 O'Donnell RD, Hordinsky JR, Madakasira S, Moise S, Warner D: A candidate automated test battery for neuropsychological screening of airmen: Design and preliminary validation. ADA247701

92-12 Revzin AM, Rasmussen PG: A new test of scanning and monitoring ability: Methods and initial results. ADA249123

92-13 Witt LA, Hellman C: Effects of subordinate feedback to the supervisor and participation in decision-making in the prediction of organizational support. ADA249125

92-14 Nakagawara VB, Loochan FK, Wood KJ: The prevalence of artificial lens implants in the civil airman population. ADA249125

92-15 Myers JG: Survey of aviation medical examiners: Information and attitudes about the pre-employment and pre-appointment drug testing program. ADA249124

92-16 Myers JG: A longitudinal examination of applicants to the air traffic supervisory identification and development program. ADA251879

92-17 Witt LA: Organizational politics, participation in decision-making, and job satisfaction. ADA251878

92-18 Wilcox BC, England HM Jr, McLean GA: Inward contaminant leakage tests of the S-Tron Corporation emergency escape breathing device. ADA251888

92-19 Teague SM, Hordinsky JR: Tolerance of beta blocked hypertensives during orthostatic and altitude stress. ADA249904

92-20 Gowdy V, DeWeese R: Evaluation of head impact kinematics for passengers seated behind interior walls. ADA252651

92-21	Witt LA: Procedural justice, occupational identification, and organizational commitment. ADA252493
92-22	England HM Jr, Wilcox BC Jr, McLean GA: Comparisons of molecular sieve oxygen concentrators for potential medical use aboard commercial aircraft. ADA253648
92-23	White VL, Canfield DV, Hordinsky JR: The identification and quantitation of triamterene in blood and urine from a fatal aircraft accident. ADA254550
92-24	Canfield DV, Kupiec TC, Huffine EF: Postmortem alcohol production in fatal aircraft accidents. ADA254680
92-25	Huffine EF, Canfield DV: Enhancement of drug detection and identification by use of various derivatizing reagents on GC-FTIR analysis. ADA254679
92-26	Manning CA, Broach D: Identifying ability requirements for operators of future automated air traffic control systems. ADA256615
92-27	McLean GA, Chittum CB, Funkhouser GE, Fairlie GW, Folk EW: Effects of seating configuration and number of type III exits on emergency aircraft evacuation. ADA255754
92-28	Mertens HW, Milburn NJ: Performance of color-dependent tasks of air traffic control specialists as a function of type and degree of color vision deficiency. ADA255794
92-29	Mertens HW, Milburn NJ: Validity of clinical color vision tests for air traffic control specialists. ADA258219
92-30	Della Rocco PS, Milburn N, Mertens H: Comparison of performance on the Shipley Institute of Living scale, air traffic control specialist selection test, and FAA Academy screen. ADA259249
92-31	OU Vortac, Edwards MB, Jones JP, Manning CA, Rotter AJ: En route air traffic controllers' use of flight progress strips: A graph-theoretic analysis. ADA259062

1993

93-1	Rodgers MD, Drechsler GK: Conversion of the CTA, Inc, en route operations concepts database into a formal sentence outline job task taxonomy. ADA261921
93-2	Collins WE: A review of civil aviation propeller-to-person accidents: 1980-1989. ADA260695
93-3	Antuñano MJ: Index of international publications in aerospace medicine. ADA262908
93-4	Schroeder DJ, Broach D, Young WC: Contribution of personality to the prediction of success in initial air traffic control specialist training. ADA264699
93-5	Galaxy Scientific Corporation: Human factors in aviation maintenance - Phase Two progress report. ADA264367
93-6	Wilcox B Jr, McLean G, England H Jr: Comparison of portable crewmember protective breathing equipment (CPBE) designs. ADA265362
93-7	Sanders DC, Endecott BR, Ritter RM, Chaturvedi AK: Variations of time-to-incapacitation and carboxyhemoglobin values in rats exposed to two carbon monoxide concentrations. ADA266109
93-8	Chaturvedi AK, Endecott BR, Ritter RM, Sanders DC: Variations in time-to-incapacitation and blood cyanide values for rats exposed to two hydrogen cyanide gas concentrations. ADA265924
93-9	Rodgers MD, Blanchard RE: Accident proneness: A research review. ADA266032
93-10	Young JW: Head and face anthropometry of adult US citizens. ADA268661
93-11	Nakagawara VB, Wood KJ: Aviation accident risk for airmen with aphakia and artificial lens implants. ADA268389
93-12	Rodgers MD: SATORI: Situation assessment through the re-creation of incidents. ADA268390
93-13	Gilliland K, Schlegel RE: Readiness to perform testing: A critical analysis of the concept and current practices. ADA269397
93-14	Armenia-Cope R, Marcus JH, Gowdy RV, DeWeese RL: An assessment of the potential for neck injury due to padding of aircraft interior walls for head impact protection. ADA270509
93-15	Galaxy Scientific Corp: Human factors in aviation maintenance - Phase three, volume 1 progress report. ADA270508
93-16	Milburn NJ, Mertens HW: Validation of an inexpensive test illuminant for aeromedical color vision screening. N94-14854
93-17	Mertens HW, Milburn NJ: Validity of FAA-approved color vision tests for Class II and Class III aeromedical screening. N94-14846

93-18   Hellman CW, Witt LA: Factors associated with continuance commitment to FAA matrix teams. ADA274561

93-19   McLean GA, Smith LT, Hill TJ, Rubenstien CJ: Physiological correlates of stress-induced decrements in human perceptual performance. ADA274240

93-20   Prinzo OV, Britton TW: ATC/pilot voice communications - A survey of the literature. ADA274457

93-21   Nakagawara VB, Wood KJ, Montgomery RW: Vision impairment and corrective considerations of civil airmen. ADA275508

93-22   Rodgers MD (ed.): An examination of the operational error database for air route traffic control centers. ADA275986

1994

94-1   Collins WE, Wayda ME: Index of FAA Office of Aviation Medicine Reports: 1961 through 1993. ADA275913

94-2   Witt AW: Perceptions of organizational support and affectivity as predictors of job satisfaction. ADA277047

94-3   OU Vortac, Edwards MB, Fuller DK, Manning CA: Automation and cognition in air traffic control: An empirical investigation. ADA277057

94-4   Broach D, Brecht-Clark J: Validation of the Federal Aviation Administration air traffic control specialist pre-training screen. ADA277549

94-5   Blanchard RE, Vardaman JJ: Human factors in airway facilities maintenance: Development of a prototype outage assessment inventory. N94-26136

94-6   Schroeder DJ, Touchstone RM, Stern JA, Stoliarov N, Thackray R: Maintaining vigilance on a simulated ATC monitoring task across repeated sessions. ADA278792

94-7   Sanders DC, Chaturvedi AK, Endecott BR, Ritter RM, Vu N: Toxicity of carbon monoxide-hydrogen cyanide gas mixtures: Exposure concentration, time-to-incapacitation, carboxyhemoglobin, and blood cyanide parameters. N94-29919

94-8   Rasmussen P, Revzin A: Scanning and monitoring performance can be affected by the reinforcement values of the events being monitored. N94-29918

94-9   Broach D, Manning CA: Validity of the air traffic control specialist nonradar screen as a predictor of performance in radar-based air traffic control training. ADA279745

94-10 Garner RP, Wilcox BC, England HM, Nakagawara VB: Effects of cold exposure on wet aircraft passengers: A review. ADA280253

94-11 Marcus JE: A review of computer evacuation models and their data needs. ADA280707

94-12 Galaxy Scientific Corp: Human factors in aviation maintenance - Phase 3, Vol. 2 progress report. ADA283287

94-13 Nye LG, Schroeder DJ, Dollar CS: Relationships of Type A behavior with biographical characteristics and training performance of air traffic control specialists. ADA283813

94-14 Canfield DV, Flemig J, Hordinsky JR, Veronneau SJH: Unreported medications used in incapacitating medical conditions found in fatal civil aviation accidents. ADA284233

94-15 Nakagawara VB, Montgomery RW, Wood KJ: The applicability of commercial glare test devices in the aeromedical certification of pilot applicants. ADA284232

94-16 White VL, Canfield DV, Hordinsky JR: Elimination of quinine in two subjects after ingestion of tonic water: An exploratory study. ADA284760

94-17 Stern JA, Boyer D, Schroeder DJ: Blink rate as a measure of fatigue: A review. ADA284779

94-18 Endecott BR, Sanders DC, Chaturvedi AK: Simultaneous gas-chromatographic determination of four toxic gases generally present in combustion gas atmospheres. ADA285666

94-19 Gowdy V: The performance of child restraint devices in transport airplane passenger seats. ADA285624

94-20 Hilton Systems, Inc: Age 60 rule research, Part I: Bibliographic database. N95-13019

94-21 Hyland DT, Kay EJ, Deimler JD, Gurman EB: Age 60 rule research, Part II: Airline pilot age and performance: A review of the scientific literature. ADA286246

94-22 Kay EJ, Harris RM, Voros RS, Hillman DJ, Hyland DT, Deimler JD: Age 60 rule research, Part III: Consolidated database experiments final report. ADA286247

94-23 Hyland DT, Kay EJ, Deimler JD: Age 60 rule research, Part IV: Experimental evaluation of pilot performance. N95-13199

94-24   Holloway FA: Low-dose alcohol effects on human behavior and performance: An update on post-1984 studies. N95-14863

94-25   Williams KW, Ed: Summary proceedings of the joint industry-FAA conference on development and use of PC-based aviation training devices. N95-14917

94-26   Stern JA, Boyer D, Schroeder DJ, Touchstone RM, Stoliarov N: Blinks, saccades, and fixation pauses during vigilance task performance. ADA290600

94-27   Endsley M, Rodgers MD: Situation awareness information requirements analysis for en route air traffic control. ADA289649

1995

95-1   Collins WE: A review of civil aviation fatal accidents in which "lost/disoriented" was a cause/factor. ADA290944

95-2   Parker JF Jr, Shepherd WT: Development of an intervention program to encourage shoulder harness use and aircraft retrofit in general aviation: Phases I and II. ADA290966

95-3   Harris HC, Schroeder DJ, Collins WE: The effects of age and low doses of alcohol on compensatory tracking during angular acceleration. N95-23934

95-4   Edwards MB, Fuller DK, OU Vortac, Manning CA: The role of flight progress strips in en route air traffic control: A time-series analysis. ADA291152

95-5   Besco RO, Sangal SP, Nesthus TE, Veronneau SJH: A longevity and survival analysis for a cohort of retired airline pilots. ADA292060

95-6   Williams KW, Blanchard RE: Qualification guidelines for personal computer-based aviation training devices: Instrument rating. ADA292961

95-7   Schroeder DJ, Harris HC, Collins WE, Nesthus TE: Some performance effects of age and low blood alcohol levels on a computerized neuropsychological test. ADA292324

95-8   Chaturvedi AK, Sanders DC: Aircraft fires, smoke toxicity, and survival: An overview. ADA292919

95-9   OU Vortac, Edwards MB, Manning CA: Functions of external cues in prospective memory. ADA291932

95-10   Myers JG: Enhancing the effects of diversity awareness training: A review of the research literature. ADA293933; N95-26361

95-11   Nakagawara VB, Montgomery RW, Wood KJ: An assessment of aviation accident risk for aphakic civil airmen by class of medical certificate held and by age. ADA293407

95-12   Cruz CE, Della Rocco PS: Sleep patterns in air traffic controllers working rapidly-rotating shifts: A field study. ADA294159; N95-26204

95-13   Mertens HW, Milburn NJ, Collins WE: Practical color vision tests for air traffic control applicants: En Route, Center, and Terminal facilities. ADA294560; N95-27323

95-14   Shepherd WT, Galaxy Scientific Corp: Human factors in aviation maintenance - Phase IV progress report. N95-27696

95-15   Prinzo OV, Hendrix A, Britton TW: Development of a coding form for approach control/pilot voice communications. N95-28540

95-16   Rodgers MD, Drechsler GK: Conversion of the TRACON operations concepts database into a formal sentence outline job task taxonomy. N95-28819

95-17   Garner RP: The potential for pulmonary heat injury resulting from the activation of a cabin water spray system to fight aircraft cabin fires. N95-29224

95-18   Rodgers M (Ed): A human factors evaluation of the operational demonstration flight inspection aircraft. N95-29365

95-19   Della Rocco PS, Cruz CE: Shift work, age and performance: Investigation of the 2-2-1 shift schedule used in air traffic control facilities I: The sleep/wake cycle. N95-29261

95-20   Funkhouser GE, George MH: Alternative methods for flotation seat cushion use. N95-29448

95-21   Hartel CEJ, Hartel GF: Controller resource management-What can we learn from aircrews? ADA297386

95-22   McLean GA, George MH, Chittum CB, Funkhouser GE: Aircraft evacuations through type-III exits I: Effects of seat placement at the exit. ADA297286

95-23   Boyer DJ: The relationship among eye movements, head movements, and manual responses in a simulated air traffic control task. ADA298753

95-24   O'Donnell R: The effect of alcohol and fatigue on an FAA readiness-to-perform test. ADA299076

95-25   McLean GA, George MH: Aircraft evacuations through type-III exits II: Effects of individual subject differences. ADA299237

95-26   Chaturvedi AK, Canfield DV: Role of metabolites in aviation forensic toxicology. ADA299212

95-27   Hunter DR: Airmen research questionnaire: Methodology and overall results. ADA300583

95-28   Canfield DV, Flemig JW, Hordinsky JR, Birky M: Drugs and alcohol found in fatal civil aviation accidents between 1989 and 1993. ADA302527

95-29   Mandella JG Jr, Garner RP: An economical alternative for the secondary container used for transporting infectious disease substances. ADA302648

95-30   DeWeese RL: An experimental abdominal pressure measurement device for child ATDs. ADA302651

95-31   Layton CF, Shepherd WT: Results of a field study of the performance enhancement system: A support system for aviation safety inspectors. ADA303336

95-32   Schroeder DJ, Rosa RR, Witt LA: Some effects of 8- vs. 10-hour work schedules on the test performance/alertness of air traffic control specialists. ADA302810

1996

96-1   Collins WE, Wayda ME: Index of FAA Office of Aviation Medicine Reports: 1961 through 1995. ADA3040263

96-2   Shepherd WT, Galaxy Scientific Corp: Human factors in aviation maintenance: Phase V progress report. ADA304262

96-3   Baker SP, Lamb MW, Li G, Dodd RS: Crashes of instructional flights: Analysis of cases and remedial approaches. ADA304890

96-4   Garner RP: Performance of a continuous flow passenger oxygen mask at an altitude of 40,000 ft. N96-22217

96-5   Albright CA, Truitt TR, Barile AB, OU Vortac, Manning CA: How controllers compensate for the lack of flight progress strips. ADA305305

96-6   Morrison JE, Fotouhi CH, Broach D: A formative evaluation of the collegiate training initiative-Air Traffic Control Specialist Program. ADA305307

96-7   Marcus J: Determination of effective thoracic mass. ADA306061

96-8   Williams KW: Qualification guidelines for personal computer-based aviation training devices: Instrument rating. ADA306206

96-9   Stern JA, Boyer D, Schroeder DJ, Touchstone RM, Stoliarov N: Blinks, saccades and fixation pauses during vigilance task performance: II. Gender and time of day. ADA307024

96-10   Kanki BG (Editor), Prinzo OV (Co-Editor): Methods and metrics of voice communications. ADA307148

96-11   Marcus JH: Dummy and injury criteria for aircraft crashworthiness. ADA308948

96-12   Nakagawara VB, Coffey JD, Montgomery RW: Ophthalmic requirements and considerations for the en route air traffic control specialist: An ergonometric analysis of the visual work environment. N96-25681

96-13   Young WC, Broach D, Farmer WL: Differential prediction of FAA Academy performance on the basis of gender and written Air Traffic Control Specialist aptitude test scores. ADA308354

96-14   Kupiec TC, Canfield DV, White VL: The analysis of benzodiazepines in forensic urine samples. ADA309377

96-15   Beringer DB: Use of off-the-shelf PC-based flight simulators for aviation human factors research. ADA309237

96-16   Beringer DB, Harris HC Jr: A comparison of the effects of navigational display formats and memory aids on pilot performance. ADA309382

96-17   Canfield D, White V, Soper J, Kupiec T: A comprehensive drug screening procedure for urine using HPLC, TLC, and mass spectroscopy. ADA309962

96-18   McLean GA, George MH, Funkhouser GE, Chittum CB: Aircraft evacuations onto escape slides and platforms I: Effects of passenger motivation. ADA311257

96-19   Kirkbride LA, Jensen RS, Chubb GP, Hunter DR: Developing the personal minimums tool for managing risk during preflight go/no-go decisions. ADA313639

96-20   Prinzo OV, Maclin O: Aviation topics speech acts taxonomy (ATSAT) pc user's guide version 2.0. ADA314179

96-21   Collins WE, Dollar CS: Fatal general aviation accidents involving spatial disorientation: 1976-1992. ADA313864

96-22   Mertens HW, Milburn NJ, Collins WE: A further validation of the practical color vision test for enroute air traffic control applicants. ADA314600

96-23   Della Rocco P, Cruz C: Shift work, age, and performance: Investigation of the 2-2-1 shift schedule used in air traffic control facilities II: Laboratory performance measures. ADA315493

96-24   Bailey L, Shaw R: Flight inspection crew resource management training needs analysis. ADA316691

96-25   Veronneau SJH, Mohler SR, Pennybaker AL, Wilcox BC, Sahiar F: Survival at high altitudes: Wheel-well passengers. ADA317375

96-26   Prinzo OV, Maclin O: An analysis of approach control/pilot voice communications. ADA317528

96-27   Nakagawara VB, Wood KJ: The use of task-specific lenses by presbyopic air traffic controllers at the en route radar console. ADA320284

1997

97-1   Collins WE, Wayda ME: Index of FAA Office of Aviation Medicine Reports: 1961 through 1996. ADA322331

97-2   DeJohn CA, Veronneau SJH, Hordinsky JR: Inflight medical care: An update. ADA322708

97-3   Driskill WE, Weissmuller JJ, Quebe J, Hand DK, Dittmar MJ, Hunter DR: The use of weather information in aeronautical decision-making. ADA323543

97-4   Young WC, Broach D, Farmer WL: The effects of video game experience on computer-based Air Traffic Control Specialist, air traffic scenario test scores. ADA322774

97-5   Gilliland K, Schlegel RE: A laboratory model of Readiness-to-Perform testing: Learning rates and reliability analyses for candidate testing measures. ADA323620

97-6   Kochan JA, Jensen RS, Chubb GP, Hunter DR: A new approach to aeronautical decision-making: The expertise method. ADA323793

97-7   Nesthus TE, Garner RP, Mills SH, Wise RA: Effects of simulated general aviation altitude hypoxia on smokers and nonsmokers. ADA323899

97-8   Thompson RC, Hilton TF, Witt LA: Where the safety rubber meets the shop floor: A confirmatory model of management influence on workplace safety. ADA324677

97-9   Nesthus TE, Rush LL, Wreggit SS: Effects of mild hypoxia on pilot performance at general aviation altitudes. ADA324719

97-10   Milburn NJ, Mertens HW: Evaluation of a range of target blink amplitudes for attention-getting value in a simulated air traffic control display. ADA326465

97-11   Taylor HL, Lintern G, Hulin CL, Talleur D, Emanuel T, Phillips S: Transfer of training effectiveness of personal computer-based aviation training devices. ADA325887

97-12   Thompson RC, Hilton TF, Behn LD: Baseline assessment of the National Association of Air Traffic Specialists/Federal Aviation Administration partnership. ADA326753

97-13   Endsley MR, Rodgers MD: Distribution of attention, situation awareness, and workload in a passive air traffic control task: Implications for operational errors and automation. ADA328997

97-14   Kupiec TC, Chaturvedi AK: Stereochemical determination of selegiline metabolites in postmortem biological specimens. ADA329026

97-15   Broach D, Manning CA: Review of air traffic controller selection: An international perspective. ADA328993

97-16   Hunter DR: An evaluation of safety seminars. ADA329009

97-17   Schroeder DJ, Dollar CS: Personality characteristics of pre/post-strike air traffic control applicants. ADA328998

97-18   Marcus JH: A flexible cabin simulator. ADA328996

97-19   Broach D: Designing selection tests for the future National Airspace System architecture. ADA329231

Part I: Chronological Index

97-20 Court MC, Marcus JH: Use of object-oriented programming to simulate human behavior in emergency evacuation of an aircraft's passenger cabin. ADA329462

97-21 Salazar GJ, DeJohn CA, Hansrote RW, Key OR: Bloodborne pathogens in aircraft accident investigation. ADA340366

97-22 Gronlund SD, Dougherty MRP, Ohrt DD, Thomson GL, Bleckley MK, Bain DL, Arnell F, Manning CA: The role of memory in air traffic control. ADA340263

97-23 Driskill WE, Weissmuller JJ, Hand DK, Hunter DR: The use of weather information in aeronautical decision-making: II. ADA340406

97-24 Beringer DB, Harris HC Jr: Automation in general aviation: Two studies of pilot responses to autopilot malfunctions. ADA340243

97-25 Gilliland K, Schlegel RE, Nesthus TE: Workshift and antihistamine effects on task performance. ADA340510

1998

98-1 Collins WE, Wayda ME: Index of FAA Office of Aviation Medicine Reports: 1961 through 1997. ADA339254

98-2 McLean GA, Chittum CB: Performance demonstrations of zinc sulfide and strontium aluminate photoluminescent floor proximity escape path marking systems. ADA339339

98-3 McLean GA, Palmerton DA, Chittum CB, George M. H, Funkhouser GE. Inflatable escape slide beam and girt strength tests: Support for revision of Technical Standard Order C-69b. ADA339410

98-4 Wolf MB, Garner RP: Effect of an airplane cabin water spray system on human thermal behavior: A theoretical study using a 25-node model of thermoregulation. ADA339365

98-5 Canfield DV, Smith MD, Adams HJ, Houston ER: Selection of an internal standard for postmortem ethanol analysis. ADA339340

98-6 Jensen RS, Guilkey JE, Hunter DR: An evaluation of pilot acceptance of the personal minimums training program for risk management. ADA340338

98-7 Driskill WE, Weissmuller JJ, Quebe J, Hand DK.; and Hunter DR: Evaluating the decision-making skills of general aviation pilots. ADA341118

98-8 Thompson RC, Agen RA, Broach DM: Differential training needs and abilities at air traffic control towers: Should all controllers be trained equally? ADA340829

98-9 Wreggit SS, Marsh DK II Cockpit integration of GPS: Initial assessment-menu formats and procedures. ADA341122

98-10 Sanders DC, Chaturvedi AK, Hordinsky JR, Aeromedical aspects of melatonin-An overview. ADA341726

98-11 Gowdy RV, DeWeese R: Evaluation of improved restraint systems for parachutists. ADA342643

98-12 Williams KW: GPS Design considerations: Displaying nearest airport information. ADA346043

98-13 Shehab RL, Schlegel RE, Palmerton DA: A human factors perspective on human external loads. ADA350729

98-14 Rodgers MD, Mogford RH, Mogford LS: The relationship of sector characteristics to operational errors. ADA350717

98-15 Mills SH: The combination of flight count and control time as a new metric of air traffic control activity. ADA350504

98-16 Gronlund SD, Ohrt DD, Dougherty MRP, Perry JL, Manning CA: Aircraft importance and its potential relevance to situation awareness. ADA350417

98-17 Prinzo OV: An analysis of voice communication in a simulated approach control environment. ADA350523

98-18 Chaturvedi AK, Vu NT, Ritter RM, Canfield DV: DNA profiling as an adjunct quality control/quality assurance in forensic toxicology. ADA379287

98-19 Cosper DK, McLean GA: Analysis of ditching and water survival training programs of major airframe manufacturers and airlines. PB99146839XSP

98-20 Prinzo OV, Lieberman P, Pickett E: An acoustic analysis of ATC communication. ADA353962

98-21 Canfield DV, Smith MD, Ritter RM, Chaturvedi AK: Preparation of carboxyhemoglobin standards and calculation of spectrophotometric quantitation constants. ADA379272

98-22 Broach D: Summative evaluation of the collegiate training initiative for air traffic control specialists program: Progress of Minnesota Air Traffic Control Training Center graduates in en route field training. ADA355085

98-23 Broach D (Editor): Recovery of the FAA Air Traffic Control specialist workforce, 1981-1992. ADA355135

98-24 Thompson RC, Bailey LL, Farmer WL: Predictors of perceived empowerment: An initial assessment. ADA355185

98-25 Nakagawara VB, Wood KJ: The aeromedical certification of photorefractive keratectomy in civil aviation: A reference guide. ADA382812

98-26 Durso FT, Truitt TR, Hackworth CA, Albright CA, Bleckley MK, Manning CA: Reduced flight progress strips in en route ATC mixed environments. ADA382818

98-27 Garner RP, Murphy RE, Hudgins CB, Mandella JG Jr: Performance of a portable oxygen breathing system at 25,000 feet altitude. ADA357729

98-28 Wickens CD, Ververs PM: Allocation of attention with head-up displays. ADA359344

1999

99-1 Collins WE, Wayda ME: Index of FAA Office of Aviation Medicine Reports: 1961 through 1998. ADA360592

99-2 Della Rocco PS, (Editor): The role of shift work and fatigue in air traffic control operational errors and incidents. ADA360730

99-3 Durso FT, Hackworth CA, Truitt TR, Crutchfield J, Nikolic D, Manning CA: Situation awareness as a predictor of performance in en route air traffic controllers. ADA360807

99-4 Garner RP: Concepts providing for physiological protection after aircraft cabin decompression in the altitude range of 60,000 to 80,000 feet above sea level. ADA360727

99-5 Gowdy V, George M, McLean GA: comparison of buckle release timing for push-button and lift-latch belt buckles. ADA360725

99-6 Nakagawara VB, Wood KJ, Montgomery RW: Refractive surgery in the civil airman population by class of medical certificate and by aviation occupation. ADA361329

99-7 Rakovan L, Wiggins MW, Jensen RS, Hunter DR: A survey of pilots on the dissemination of safety information. ADA361233

99-8 Milburn NJ, Mertens HW: Optimizing blink parameters for highlighting an air traffic control situation display. ADA316258

99-9 Joseph K, Jahns D, Nendick M, St. George R: A usability survey of GPS avionics equipment: Some prelimary findings. ADA362193

99-10 McLean GA, George MH, Funkhouser GE, Chittum CB: Aircraft evacuations onto escape slides and platforms II: Effects of exit size. ADA362480

99-11 Chaturvedi AK: First seven years (1991-1998) of the FAA's postmortem forensic toxicology proficiency testing program. ADA362556

99-12 Pounds J, Bailey LL: Cognitive style and learning: Performance of Adaptors and Innovators in a novel dynamic task. ADA363458

99-13 Williams KW: GPS user-interface design problems. ADA363331

99-14 Vu NT, Chaturvedi AK, Canfield DV: Urinary genotyping for DQA1 and PM loci using PCR-based amplification: Effects of sample volume, storage temperature, preservatives, and aging on DNA extraction and typing. ADA363461

99-15 Lewis RJ, Huffine EF, Chaturvedi AK, Canfield DV, Mattson J: Formation of an interfering substance, 3,4-dimethyl-5-phenyl-1,3-oxazolidine, during a pseudoephedrine urinalysis. ADA363777

99-16 Broach D, Farmer WL, Young WC: Differential prediction of FAA Academy performance on the basis of race and written Air Traffic Control Specialist aptitude test scores. ADA363587

99-17 Joseph KM, Thompson RC, Bailey LL, Williams CA, Worley JA, Schroeder DJ: The influence of ergonomics interventions on employee stress and physical symptoms. ADA364891

99-18 Heil MC: An investigation of the relationship between chronological age and job performance for incumbent Air Traffic Control Specialists. ADA364893

99-19 Behn LD, Thompson RC, Hilton TF: Follow-up assessment of the Federal Aviation Administration's Logistics Center safety climate. ADA365569

99-20 Gilliland K, Schlegel RE, Nesthus TE: Effects of antihistamine, age, and gender on task performance. ADA366860

99-21 Morrow DG, Prinzo OV: Improving pilot/ATC voice communication in General Aviation. ADA367894

99-22 Milke RM, Becker JT, Lambrou P, Harris HC, Schroeder DJ: The effects of age and practice on aviation-relevant concurrent task performance. ADA367887

99-23 Heil MC: The relationship between ATCS age and cognitive test performance. ADA368670

99-24 Bailey LL, Broach DM, Thompson, RC, Enos RJ: Controller Teamwork Evaluation and Assessment Methodology: A Scenario Calibration Study. ADA370417

99-25 Worley JA, Bailey LL, Thompson RC, Joseph KM, Williams CA: Organizational communication and trust in the context of technology change. ADA370769

99-26 Williams KW: GPS user-interface design problems: II. ADA363331

99-27 Thompson RC, Bailey LL, Joseph KM, Worley JA, Williams CA: Organizational change: Effects of fairness perceptions on cynicism. ADA371588

99-28 Sirevaag EJ, Rohrbaugh JW, Stern JA, Vedeniapin AB, Packingham KD, LaJonchere CM: Multi-dimensional characterizations of operator state: A validation of oculomotor metrics.

99-29 Soper JW, Chaturvedi AK, Canfield DV: Prevalence of chlorpheniramine in aviation accident pilot fatalities, 1991-1996. ADA372538

99-30 Hynes MK: Frequency and costs of transport airplane precautionary emergency evacuations. ADA372580

2000

00-1 Collins WE, Wayda ME: Index to FAA Office of Aviation Medicine Reports: 1961 through 1999. ADA373794

00-2 Manning CA (Editor): Measuring Air Traffic Controller Performance in a High-Fidelity Simulation. ADA373813

00-3 Hilton TF, Hart IS, Farmer WL, Thompson JJ, Behn LD: The FAA Health Awareness Program: Results of the 1998 customer service assessment survey. ADA373761

00-4 Joseph KM, Jahns DW: Enhancing GPS receiver certification by examining pilot-performance databases. PB2001102907

00-5 Truitt TR, Durso FT, Crutchfield JM, Moertl P, Manning CA: Reduced posting and marking of flight progress strips for en route air traffic control. PB2001102908

00-6 Garner RP, Murphy RE, Donnelly SS, Thompson KE, Geiwitz KL: Testing the structural integrity of the Air Force's Emergency Passenger Oxygen System at altitude. PB2001102909

00-7 Shappell SA, Weigmann DA: The Human Factors Analysis and Classification System-HFACS. PB2001102910

00-8 Williams KW: Comparing text and graphics in navigation display design. ADA375445

00-9 Chaturvedi AK, Smith DR, Canfield DV: Blood carbon monoxide and cyanide concentrations in the fatalities of fire and non-fire associated civil aviation accidents. PB2001102911

00-10 Della Rocco PS, Comperatore C, Caldwell L, Cruz CE: The effects of napping on night shift performance. PB2001102912

00-11 Hynes MK: Evacuee injuries and demographics in transport airplane precautionary emergency evacuations. PB2001102913

00-12 Heil MC, Agnew BO: The effects of previous computer experience on Air Traffic-Selection and Training (AT-SAT) test performance. ADA377228

00-13 DeJohn CA, Veronneau SJH, Wolbrink AM, Larcher JG: The evaluation of in-flight medical care aboard selected U.S. air carriers: 1996 to 1997. ADA377878

00-14 Thompson RC, Joseph KM, Bailey LL, Worley JA, Williams CA: Organizational change: An assessment of trust and cynicism. PB2001102914

00-15 Russell CJ, Dean MA, Broach DM: Guidelines for bootstrapping validity coefficients in ATCS selection research. ADA379430

00-16 Vu NT, Chaturvedi AK, Canfield DV, Soper JW, Kupfer DM, Roe BA: DNA-based detection of ethanol-producing microorganisms in postmortem blood and tissues by polymerase chain reaction. ADA379226

00-17 Thompson RC, Bailey LL: Age and attitudes in the air traffic control specialist workforce: An initial investigation. ADA379286

00-18 Nakagawara VB, Veronneau SJH: A unique contact lens-related airline aircraft accident. ADA379287

00-19 Nakagawara VB, Wood KJ, Montgomery RW: Refractive surgery in aircrew members who fly for scheduled and non-scheduled civilian airlines. PB2001102915

00-20 Lewis RJ, Johnson RD, Blank CL: A novel method for the determination of sildenafil (Viagra®) and its metabolite in postmortem specimens using LC/MS/MS and LC/MS/MS. PB2001102916

00-21 Canfield DV, Hordinsky J, Millett DP, Endecott B, Smith D: Prevalence of drugs and alcohol in fatal civil aviation accidents between 1994 and 1998. ADA379272

00-22 Canfield DV, Chaturvedi AK, Boren HK, Veronneau SJH, White VL: Abnormal glucose levels found in transportation accidents. PB2001102917

00-23 Nakagawara VB, Montgomery RW: Gender differences in a refractive surgery population of civilian aviators. PB2001102918

00-24 Pfleiderer EM: Multidimensional scaling analysis of controllers' perceptions of aircraft performance characteristics. ADA382823

00-25 Bailey L, Thompson R: The effects of performance feedback on air traffic control team coordination: A simulation study. ADA382812

00-26 Schvaneveldt R, Beringer DB, Lamonica J, Tucker R, Nance C: Priorities, organization, and sources of information accessed by pilots in various phases of flight. ADA382818

00-27 Naff KC, Thompson RC: The impact of teams on the climate for diversity in government: The FAA experience. ADA382809

00-28 Bailey LL, Peterson LM, Williams KW, Thompson RC: Controlled flight into terrain: A study of pilot perspectives in Alaska. ADA382989

00-29 Lewis RJ, Southern TL, Cardona PS, Canfield DV, Garber M: Distribution of butalbital in biological fluids and tissues. PB2001102919

00-30 Mills, SH: The computerized analysis of ATC tracking data for an operational evaluation of CDTI/ADS-B technology. ADA385812

00-31 Williams K: Impact of aviation highway-in-the-sky displays on pilot situation awareness. ADA384535

00-32 Fiedler ER, Della Rocco PS, Schroeder DJ, Nguyen K: The relationship between aviators' home-based stress to work stress and self-perceived performance. ADA384889

00-33 Nicholas J, Copeland K, Duke F, Friedberg W, O'Brien K: Galactic cosmic radiation exposure of pregnant aircrew members II. ADA385597

00-34 Chaturvedi AK, Smith DR, Canfield DV: A fatality caused by hydrogen sulfide produced from an accidental transfer of sodium hydrosulfide into a tank containing iron sulfate and sulfuric acid. ADA385303

2001

01-1 Collins WE, Wayda ME: Index to FAA Office of Aviation Medicine Reports: 1961 Through 2000. ADA389987

01-2 McLean GA: Access to egress: A meta-analysis of the factors that control emergency evacuation through the transport airplane Type-III overwing exit. PB2001104655

01-3 Wiegmann DA, Shappell SA: A human error analysis of commercial aviation accidents using the Human Factors Analysis and Classification System (HFACS). ADA 387808

01-4 Farmer WL, Thompson RC, Heil SKR, Heil MC: Latent trait theory analysis of changes in item response anchors. ADA388056

01-5 Ramos RA, Heil MC, Manning CA: Documentation of validity for the ATSAT computerized test battery, Volume I. ADA389852

01-6 Ramos RA, Heil MC, Manning CA: Documentation of validity for the ATSAT computerized test battery, Volume II. ADA389898

01-7 Nakagawara VB, Montgomery RW: Laser pointers: Their potential affects on vision and aviation safety. ADA392899

01-8 Prinzo OV: Datalinked pilot reply time on controller workload and communication in a simulated terminal option. ADA391932

Part I: Chronological Index

01-9   Prinzo OV: Innovations in pilot visual acquisition of traffic: New phraseology for Air Traffic Control operational communication.

01-10   Manning CA, Mills SH, Fox CM, Pfleiderer EM, Mogilka H: Investigating the validity of performance and objective workload evaluation research (POWER). ADA392932

01-11   Fiedler ER, Orme DR, Mills W, Patterson JC: Assessment of head-injured aircrew: Comparison of FAA and USAF procedures. ADA392805

01-12   White VL, Chaturvedi AK, Canfield DV, Garber M: Association of postmortem blood hemoglobin Alc levels with diabetic conditions in aviation accident pilot fatalities. ADA392942

01-13   Williams KW: Qualification guidelines for personal computerbased aviation training devices: Private pilot certificate. ADA396322

01-14   Nakagawara VB, Montgomery RW, Wood KJ: Aviation accidents and incidents associated with the use of ophthalmic devices by civilian pilots. ADA396122

01-15   Antuñano MJ, Wade K: Index of International Publications in Aerospace Medicine. ADA262908

01-16   Gronlund SD, Dougherty MRP, Durso FT, Canning JM, Mills SH: Planning in air traffic control. PB2002103420

01-17   Mejdal S, McCauley ME: Human factors design guidelines for multifunction displays. ADA399354

01-18   Corbett CL: Caring for precious cargo, Part I: Emergency aircraft evacuations with infants onto inflatable escape slides. ADA398987

01-19   Peterson LM, Bailey LL: Controller-to-controller communication and coordination taxonomy. PB2002103423

01-20   Bailey LL, Willems BF, Peterson LM: The effects of workload and decision support automation on enroute R-side and D-side communication exchanges. ADA399353

2002

02-1   Gronlund SD, Canning JM, Moertl PM, Johansson J, Dougherty MRP, Mills SH: An information tool for planning in air traffic control. ADA399806

02-2   Mills SH, Pfleiderer EM, Manning CA: POWER: Objective activity and taskload assessment in en route air traffic control. ADA401922

02-3   Uhlarik J, Comerford DA: A review of situation awareness literature relevant to pilot surveillance functions. ADA401774

02-4   Manning CA, Mills SH, Fox C, Pfleiderer E, Mogilka HJ: Using air traffic control taskload measures and communication events to predict subjective workload. ADA401923

02-5   Prinzo OV: Automatic dependent surveillance/broadcast-cockpit display of traffic information: Innovations in pilot-managed departures. PB2002107795

02-6   Nakagawara VB, Wood KJ, Montgomery RW: Contact lens use in the civil airman population. ADA404962

02-7   Beringer DB: Applying performance-controlled systems, fuzzy logic, and fly-by-wire controls to general aviation. ADA405731

02-8   Cruz C, Detwiler C, Nesthus T, Boquet A: A laboratory comparison of clockwise and counter-clockwise rapidly rotating shift schedules, Part I: Sleep. ADA402842

02-9   Broach D, Dollar C: Relationship of employee attitudes and supervisor-controller ration to en route operational error rates. ADA405141

02-10   Nakagawara VB, Montgomery RW, Wood KJ: The aviation accident experience of civilian airmen with refractive surgery. ADA428733

02-11   DeWeese R, Gowdy RV: Human factors associated with the certification of airplane seats: Seat belt adjustment and release. ADA404285

02-12   Pounds J, Isaac A: Development of an FAA-EUROCONTROL technique for the analysis of human error in ATM. ADA405379

02-13   Cruz C, Boquet A, Detwiler C, Nesthus T: A laboratory comparison of clockwise and counter-clockwise rapidly rotating shift schedules, Part II: Performance. ADA405385

02-14   Chaturvedi AK, Smith DR, Soper JW, Canfield DV: Characteristics and toxicological processing of postmortem pilot specimens from fatal civil aviation accidents. ADA405378

02-15   Lewis RJ, Johnson RD, Canfield DV: An accurate method for the determination of carbon monoxide in postmortem blood using GC/TCD. ADA408214

02-16   McLean GA, Corbett CL, Larcher KG, McDown JR, Palmerton DA, Porter KA, Shaftstall RM, Odom RS: Access-to-Egress: Interactive effects of factors that control the emergency evacuation of naïve passengers through the transport airplane Type-III overwing exit. ADA408009

02-17   Hunter D: Risk perception and risk tolerance in aircraft pilots. ADA40799

02-18   Bailey LL, Willems BF: The moderator effects of taskload on the interplay between en route intra-sector team communications, situation awareness, and mental workload. ADA408021

02-19   Roy KM, Beringer DB: General aviation pilot performance following unannounced in-flight loss of vacuum system and associated instruments in simulated instrument meteorological conditions. ADA408027

02-20   Boquet A, Cruz C, Nesthus TE, Detwiler C, Knecht W, Holcomb K: A laboratory comparison of clockwise and counter-clockwise rapidly rotating shift schedule, Part III: Effects on core body temperatures and neuroendocrine measures. ADA409994

02-21   Williams KW, Yost A, Holland J, Tyler RR: Assessment of advanced cockpit displays for GA aircraft: The Capstone Program. ADA409997

02-22   Moertl PM, Canning JM, Gronlund SD, Dougherty MRP, Johansson J, Mills SH: Aiding planning in air traffic control: An experimental investigation of the effects of perceptual information integration. ADA409992

02-23   Goldman SM, Fiedler ER, King RE: General aviation maintenance-related accidents: A review of 10 years of NTSB data. ADA409385

02-24   Heil MC, Detwiler CA, Agen RA, Williams CA, Agnew BO, King RE: The effects of practice and coaching on the Air Traffic Selection and Training Battery. ADA409734

2003

03-1   Collins WE, Wayda ME: Index of FAA Office of Aerospace Medicine Reports: 1961 through 2002. ADA410971

03-2   Joseph KM, Domino D, Battisie V, Bone RS, Olmos BO: A summary of flightdeck observer data from SafeFlight 21 OpEval-2. ADA413898

03-3   Taylor HL, Talleur DA, Bradshaw GL, Eanuel TW Jr., Rantanen E, Hulin CL, Lendrum L: Effectiveness of personal computers to meet recency of experience requirements. ADA413334

03-4   Shappell SA Wiegmann DA: A human error analysis of general aviation controlled flight into terrain accidents occurring between 1990-1998. ADA417230

03-5   Uhlarik J, Comerford DA: Information requirements for traffic awareness in a free-flight environment: An application of the FAIT Analysis. ADA413832

03-6   Nakagawara VB, Wood KJ, Montgomery RW: Natural sunlight and its association to aviation accidents: Frequency and prevention. ADA417208

03-7   Akin A, Chaturvedi AK: Prevalence of selective serotonin reuptake inhibitors in pilot fatalities of civil aviation accidents, 1990-2001. ADA423836

03-8   Pfleiderer EM: Development of an empirically based index of aircraft mix. ADA417231

03-9   Gowdy V, DeWeese R: Human factors associated with the certification of airplane passenger seats: Life preserver retrieval. ADA417209

03-10   Hackworth CA, Peterson LM, Jack DG, Williams CA, Hodges BE: Examining hypoxia: A survey of pilots' experiences and perspectives on altitude training. ADA417131

03-11   Hackworth CA, King SJ, Detwiler CA: The employee attitude survey 2000: Perspectives on its process and utility. ADA417166

03-12   Nakagawara VB, Montgomery RW, Dillard A, McLin L, Connor CW: Effects of laser illumination on operational and visual performance of pilots conducting terminal operations. ADA423865

Part I: Chronological Index

03-13 Prinzo OV, Hendrix AM: Automatic dependent surveillance-broadcast/cockpit display of traffic information: Pilot use of the approach spacing application. ADA423864

03-14 Dollar C, Broach D, Schroeder D: Personality characteristics of air traffic control specialists as predictors of disability retirement. ADA424266

03-15 Corbett CL, McLean GA, Whinnery JE: Access-to-Egress II: Subject management and injuries in a study of emergency evacuation through the Type-III exit. ADA423728

03-16 Friedberg W, Copeland K: What aircrews should know about their occupational exposure to ionizing radiation. ADA423589

03-17 Williams K, Ball J: Usability and effectiveness of advanced general aviation cockpit displays for instrument flight procedures. ADA423591

03-18 Johnson RD, Lewis RJ, Canfield DV, Blank, CL: Ethanol origin in postmortem urine: An LC/MS determination of serotonin metabolites. ADA423727

03-19 Pounds J, Ferrante A: FAA strategies for identifying and reducing operational error causal factors. ADA423665

03-20 King RE, Retzlaff PD, Detwiler C, Schroeder DJ, Broach D: Use of personality assessment measures in the selection of air traffic control specialists. ADA423269

03-21 Pounds J, Isaac A: Validation of the JANUS technique: Causal factors of human error in operational incidents. ADA423271

03-22 Chaturvedi AK, Cardona PS, Soper JW, Canfield DV: Distribution and optical purity of methamphetamine found in toxic concentration in a civil aviation accident pilot fatality. ADA423609

03-23 Lewis RJ, Johnson RD, Angier MK, Ritter RM, Drilling HS, Williams SD: Analysis of cocaine, its metabolites, prolysis products, and ethanol adducts in postmortem fluids and tissues using Zymark automated solid-phase extractions and gas chromatography-mass spectrometry. ADA423349

03-24 Cardona PS, Chaturvedi AK, Soper JW, Canfield DV: Simultaneous determination of cocaine, cocaethylene, and their possible pentafluoropropylated metabolites and pryolysis products by gas chromatography/mass spectrometry. ADA423601

2004

04-1 Vu NT, Zhu H, Owuor ED, Huggins ME, White VL, Chaturvedi AK, Canfield DV, Whinnery JE: Isolation of RNA from peripheral blood cells: A validation study for molecular diagnostics by microassay and kinetic RTC-PCR assays— Application in aerospace medicine. ADA428748

04-2 McLean GA, Corbett CL: Access-to-egress III: Repeated measurement of factors that control the emergency evacuation of passengers through the transport airplane Type-III overwing exit. ADA423562

04-3 Garner RP, Ultrecht JS: Performance criteria for development of extended use protective breathing equipment. ADA423233

04-4 Johnson RD, Lewis RJ, Angier MK, Vu NT: The formation of ethanol in postmortem tissues. ADA423300

04-5 Beringer DB, Ball JD: The effects of NEXRAD graphical data resolution and direct weather viewing on pilot's judgments of weather severity and their willingness to continue a flight. ADA423239

04-6 Nakagawara VB, Montgomery RW, Wood KJ: Demographics and vision restrictions in civilian pilots: Clinical implications. ADA423237

04-7 Garner RP, Wong KL, Ericson SC, Baker AJ, Orzechowski JA: CFD validation for contaminant transport in aircraft cabin ventilation flow fields. ADA423999

04-8 Broach D: Methodological issues in the study of airplane accident rates by pilot age: Effects of accident and pilot inclusion criteria and analytic strategy. ADA423237

04-9 Nakagawara VB, Montgomery RW, Dillard AE, McLin LN, Connor CW: The effects of laser illumination on operational and visual performance of pilots during final approach. ADA425392

04-10 Milburn NJ: A historical review of color vision standards for automated flight service station air traffic control specialists. ADA426278

04-11   Prinzo OV: Automatic Dependent Surveillance-Broadcast/Cockpit Display of Traffic Information: Innovations in aircraft navigation on the airport surface. ADA427908

04-12   McLean GA, Palmerton DA, Corbett CL, Larcher KG, McDown JR: Simulated evacuations into water. ADA427908

04-13   Johnson RD, Lewis RJ, Canfield DV, Dubowski KM, Blank CL: Accurate assignment of ethanol origin in postmortem urine: A case study. ADA427914

04-14   Milburn NJ, Mertens HW: Predictive validity of the aviation lights test for testing pilots with color vision deficiencies. ADA428358

04-15   Angier MK, Lewis RJ, Chaturvedi AK, Canfield DV: Gas chromatographic/mass spectrometric differentiation of atenolol, metoprolol, propanolol, and an interfering metabolite product of metoprolol. ADA428964

04-16   DeJohn CA, Wolbrink AM, Larcher JG: In-flight medical incapacitation and impairment of U.S. airline pilots: 1993 to 1998. ADA428688

04-17   Xing J: Measures of information complexity and the implications for automation design. ADA428690

04-18   DeWeese R, Moorcroft D: Evaluation of a head injury criteria component test device. ADA428692

04-19   McLean GA, Cosper DK: Availability of passenger safety information for improved survival in aircraft accidents. ADA372580

04-20   Williams KW, Ball JD: Usability and effectiveness of advanced general aviation cockpit displays for visual flight procedures. ADA423591

04-21   Dollar CS, Schroeder DJ: A longitudinal study of Myers-Briggs personality types in air traffic controllers. ADA460091

04-22   Hackworth CA, Cruz CE, Goldman S, Jack DG, King SJ, Twohig P: Employee attitudes within the Federal Aviation Administration. ADA460092

04-23   Hackworth CA, Cruz CE, Jack DG, Goldman S, King SJ: Employee attitudes within the air traffic organization. ADA460936

04-24   Williams K: A summary of unmanned aircraft accident/incident data: Human factors implications. ADA460102

2005

05-1   Collins WE, Wayda ME, Wade K: Index to FAA Office of Aerospace Medicine Reports: 1961 through 2004. ADA460101

05-2   Corbett CL: Caring for precious cargo, Part II: Behavioral techniques for emergency aircraft evacuations with infants through the Type III overwing exit. ADA460057

05-3   Collins WE, Wade KJ: A milestone of aeromedical research contributions to civil aviation safety: The 1000th report in the CARI/OAM series. ADA460106

05-4   Xing J, Manning CA: Complexity and automation displays of air traffic control: Literature review and analysis. ADA460107

05-5   Bailey L, Schroeder DJ, Pounds J: The Air Traffic Control Operational Errors Severity Index: An initial evaluation. ADA460573

05-6   Broach D: Review of the scientific basis for the mandatory separation of an ATCS at Age 56. ADA460056

05-7   Knecht WR, Harris H, Shappell S: The influence of visibility, cloud ceiling, financial incentive, and personality factors on general aviation pilots' willingness to take off into marginal weather: Part I. The data and preliminary conclusions. ADA460734

05-8   Wang SM, Lewis RJ, Canfield D, Lio TL, Liu RH: Enantiomeric analysis of epedrines and norephedrines. ADA460874

05-9   Canfield DV, Chaturvedi AK, Dubowski KM: Interpretation of carboxyhemoglobin and cyanide concentrations in relation to aviation accidents. ADA460835

05-10   Johnson RD, Lewis RJ: Simultaneous quantitation of atenolol, metoprolol, and propranolol in biological matrices via LC/MS. ADA460843

05-11   Johnson RD, Lewis RJ, Hattrup RA: Poppy seed consumption or opiate use: The determination of thebaine and opiates of abuse in postmortem fluids and tissues. ADA460858

Part I: Chronological Index

05-12 Beringer DB, Harris HC Jr: A comparison of baseline hearing thresholds between pilots and non-pilots and the effects of engine noise. ADA460838

05-13 King SJ, Cruz CE, Jack DG, Thomas S, Hackworth CA: 2003 Employee Attitude Survey: Analysis of employee comments. ADA460830

05-14 Copeland K, Sauer HH, Friedberg W: Solar radiation alert system. ADA460733

05-15 Knecht WR: Pilot willingness to take off into marginal weather, Part II: antecedent overfitting with forward stepwise logistic regression. ADA460841

05-16 Pfleiderer EM: Relationship of the aircraft mix index with performance and objective workload evaluation research measures and controllers' subjective complexity ratings. ADA460790

05-17 Palmerton D: Fatality and injury rates for two types of rotorcraft accidents. ADA460769

05-18 Garner RP, Mandella JG Jr: Reliability of the gas supply in the air force emergency passenger oxygen system. ADA460831

05-19 Prinzo OV: Terminal radar approach control: Measures of voice communications system performance. ADA460833

05-20 Chaturvedi AK, Craft KJ, Canfield DV, Whinnery JE: Epidemiology of toxicological factors in civil aviation accident pilot fatalities, 1999-2003. ADA460798

05-21 Nakagawara VB, Montgomery RW, Good GW: Medical surveillance programs for aircraft maintenance personnel performing nondestructive inspection and testing. ADA460862

05-22 Broach D, Schroeder D: Relationship of air traffic control specialist age to en route operational errors. ADA460816

05-23 Beringer DB, Ball JD, Brennan K, Taite S: Comparison of a typical electronic attitude-direction indicator with terrain-depicting primary flight displays for performing recoveries from unknown attitudes: Using difference and equivalence tests. ADA460873

05-24 Wiegmann D, Faaborg T, Boquet A, Detwiler C, Holcomb K, Shappell S: Human error and general aviation accidents: A comprehensive, fine-grained analysis using HFACS. ADA460866

05-25 Scarborough A, Bailey LL, Pounds J: Examining ATC operational errors using the Human Factors Analysis and Classification System. ADA460879

2006

06-1 Antuñano MJ, Baisden DL, Davis J, Hastings J, Jennings R, Jones D, Jordan JL, Mohler S, Ruehle C, Salazar GJ, Silberman WS, Scarpa P, Tilton FE, Whinnery JE: Guidance for medical screening of commercial aerospace passengers. ADA460819

06-2 Xing J, Schroeder D: Re-examination of color vision standards, Part I: Status of color use in ATC displays and demography of color-deficit controllers. ADA460875

06-3 Johnson RD, Lewis RJ: Identification of Sildenafil (Viagra®) and Its metabolite (UK-103,320) in six aviation fatalities. ADA460880

06-4 Goldman SM, Manning C, Pfleiderer E: Static sector characteristics and operational errors. ADA460882

06-5 Johnson RD, Lewis RJ, Whinnery JE, Forster EM: Aeromedical aspects of aircraft-assisted pilot suicides in the U.S., 1993-2002. ADA460820

06-6 Xing J, Schroeder DJ: Reexamination of color vision standards, Part II. A computational method to assess the effect of color deficiencies in using ATC displays. ADA463063

06-7 Detwiler C, Hackworth C, Holcomb K, Boquet A, Pfleiderer E, Wiegmann D, Shappell, S: Beneath the tip of the iceberg: A human factors analysis of general aviation accidents in Alaska vs. the rest of the United States. ADA460891

06-8 Williams KW: Human factors implications of unmanned aircraft accidents: Flight control problems. ADA460892

06-9 Nakagarwara VB, Wood KJ, Montgomery RW: New refractive surgery procedures and their implications for aviation safety. ADA460896

06-10 Shaffstall RM, Garner RP, Bishop J, Cameron-Landis L, Eddington DL, Hau G, Spera S, Mielnik T, Thomas JA: Vaporized hydrogen peroxide (VHP®) decontamination of a section of a Boeing 747 cabin. ADA460897

06-11 Xing J: Reexamination of color vision standards, Part III: Analysis of the effect of color vision deficiencies in using ATC displays. ADA460956

06-12 Canfield DV, Salazar GJ, Lewis RJ, Whinnery JE: Comparison of pilot medical history and medications found in postmortem specimens. ADA461233

06-13 Nesthus TE, Cruz C, Hackworth C, Boquet A: An assessment of commuting risk factors for air traffic control specialists. ADA460857

06-14 Kupfer DM, Huggins M, Cassidy B, Vu N, Burian D, Canfield D: A rapid and inexpensive PCR-based STR genotyping method for identifying forensic specimens. ADA460885

06-15 Xing J: Color and visual factors in ATC displays. ADA460886

06-16 Dattel AR, King RE: Reweighing AT-SAT to mitigate group score differences. ADA461242

06-17 Johnson RD, Lewis RJ, Angier MK: The LC/MS quantitation of Vardenafil (Levitra®) in postmortem biological specimens. ADA460865

06-18 Shappell SA, Detwiler CA, Holcomb KA, Hackworth CA, Boquet AJ, Wiegmann DA: Human error and commercial aviation accidents: A comprehensive, fine-grained analysis using HFACS. ADA463865

06-19 Caldwell DC, Lewis RJ, Shaffstall RM, Johnson RD: Sublimation rate of dry ice packaged in commonly used quantities by the air cargo industry. ADA461451

06-20 Pounds J, Rodgers MD, Thompson D, Jack DG: Developing temporal markers to profile operational errors. ADA461407

06-21 Schroeder D, Bailey L, Pounds J, Manning C: A human factors review of the operational error literature. ADA461408

06-22 Xing J: Color analysis in air traffic control displays, Part I. Radar displays. ADA461409

06-23 Nakagawara VB, Wood KJ, Montgomery RW: A review of recent laser illumination events in the aviation environment. ADA461728

06-24 Shappell S, Wiegmann D: Developing a methodology for assessing safety programs targeting human error in aviation. ADA461400

06-25 Prinzo OV, Hendrix AM, Hendrix R: The outcome of ATC message complexity on pilot readback performance. ADA461355

06-26 Milburn NJ, Dobbins L, Pounds J, Goldman S: Mining for information in accident data. ADA464086

06-27 Baker AJ, Ericson SC, Orzechowski JA, Wong KL, Garner RP: Validation for CFD prediction of mass transport in an aircraft passenger cabin. ADA465914

06-28 Nakagawara VB, Montgomery RW, Wood KJ: Aircraft accidents and incidents associated with visual disturbances from bright lights during nighttime flight operations. ADA465917

06/29 Manning CM, Pfleiderer EM: Relationship of sector activity and sector complexity to air traffic controller taskload. ADA463881

06/30 Dollar C, Broach D: Comparison of intent-to-leave with actual turnover within the FAA. ADA463866

PART II: AUTHOR INDEX

A

Abbott JK — 70-4, 70-13, 72-12, 77-9, 83-12, 85-4, 86-3, 86-5
Adams HJ — 98-5
Adams T — 63-23, 63-25, 65-16, 65-28, 65-29, 65-30, 66-23
Agee FL Jr — 66-24
Agen RA — 98-8, 02-24
Agnew BO — 00-12, 02-24
Akin A — 03-7
Albright CA — 96-5, 98-26
Allen ME — TechPub#1, 64-16, 65-17, 66-1, 66-2, 68-7
Allgood MA — 70-16, 75-2, 75-13
Alluisi EA — 78-34
Anderson JA — 79-23, 80-12
Angier MK — 03-23, 04-4, 04-15, 06-17
Antuñano MJ — 93-3, 01-15, 06-1, 06-1
Armenia-Cope R — 93-14
Armstrong R — 66-17
Arnell F — 97-22
Ashby FK — 67-8
Atocknie PA — 89-10
Aul JC — 92-5
Aviation Medical Library FAA — 64-20

B

Badgley JM — 69-22
Bailey JP — 73-16, 74-9, 75-8, 77-18, 78-11
Bailey LL — 96-24, 98-24, 99-17, 99-24, 99-25, 99-27, 00-14, 00-17, 00-25, 00-28, 01-19, 01-20, 02-18, 06-21, 05-5, 05-25
Bain DL — 97-22
Baisden DL — 06-1
Baker AJ — 04-7, 06-27
Baker SP — 96-3
Balke B — 62-6, 63-6, 63-12, 63-18, 63-33, 63-34, 64-2, 64-3, 66-36
Ball JD — 03-17, 04-5, 04-20, 05-23
Bannister JR — 78-4
Barile AB — 96-5
Barnard C — 66-16
Bartanowicz RS — 86-2
Battisie V — 03-2

Baxter NE — 84-6, 90-1
Bedell RHS — 67-22
Behn LD — 97-12, 99-19, 00-3
Beiergrohslein D — 78-26
Bergey KH — 72-27
Bergin JM — 73-5
Beringer DB — 96-15, 96-16, 97-24, 00-26, 02-7, 02-19, 04-5, 05-12, 05-23
Berkley WJ — 65-5, 65-6
Berninger D — 91-16
Besco RO — 95-5
Billings CE — 72-4
Billings SM — 67-17
Birkey M — 95-28
Biron WJ — 84-1
Bishop J — 06-10
Blanchard RE — 93-9, 94-5, 95-6
Blank CL — 00-20, 03-18, 04-13
Bleckley MK — 97-22
Blethrow JG — 66-42, 70-19, 72-15, 77-11, 78-3, 79-22, 80-12
Blossom CW — 78-31
Bolding FA — 80-8
Bone RS — 03-2
Boone JO — 78-10, 78-36, 79-14, 79-21, 80-5, 80-7, 80-15, 82-2, 82-11, 82-18, 83-6, 83-9
Booze CF Jr — 68-5, 68-9, 69-11, 70-18, 72-13, 73-8, 73-10, 74-5, 75-5, 76-7, 77-10, 77-20, 78-21, 79-19, 80-8, 81-9, 81-14, 83-18, 84-3, 84-8, 85-6, 87-7, 89-2, 90-7
Boquet A — 02-8, 02-13, 02-20, 05-24, 06-7, 06-13, 06-18
Boren HK — 00-22
Bourdet NM — 71-36
Boyer D — 94-17, 94-26, 95-23, 96-9
Braden GE — 69-22, 73-1
Bradshaw GL — 03-3
Brake CM — 62-18, 63-1, 63-16, 63-22, 63-32, 65-27
Branson DM — 85-11
Brecher GA — 69-23, 70-2, 71-22, 72-8
Brecher MH — 69-23, 70-2, 71-22
Brecht-Clark J — 94-4
Brennan R — 05-23
Britton TW — 93-20, 95-15

Part II: Author Index

Author	Report Number
Broach DM	91-4, 91-11, 91-18, 92-26, 93-4, 94-4, 94-9, 96-6, 96-13, 97-4, 97-15, 97-19, 98-8, 98-22, 98-23, 99-16, 99-24, 00-15, 02-9, 03-14, 03-20, 04-8, 05-6, 05-22, 06-30
Broadhurst JL	72-30
Bruni CB	69-6, 69-16
Bryant KD	89-6
Burian D	06-14
Busby DE	77-11

C

Author	Report Number
Caldwell DC	06-19
Caldwell L	00-10
Cameron-Landis L	06-10
Canfield DV	91-12, 92-23, 92-24, 92-25, 94-14, 94-16, 95-26, 95-28, 96-14, 96-17, 98-5, 98-18, 98-21, 99-14, 99-15, 99-29, 00-9, 00-16, 00-21, 00-22, 00-29, 00-34, 01-12, 02-14, 02-15, 03-18, 03-22, 03-24, 04-1, 04-13, 04-15, 05-8, 05-9, 05-20, 06-12, 06-14
Canning JM	01-16, 02-1, 02-22
Capps MJ	Tech.Pub.#1, 64-14, 65-1, 65-2
Cardona PS	00-29, 03-22, 03-24
Carroll JJ	70-16
Cassidy B	06-14
Chandler RF	68-24, 72-27, 74-4, 76-9, 77-11, 78-6, 78-12, 78-23, 78-24, 79-17, 80-12, 82-8, 83-16
Chase RC	72-4
Chaturvedi AK	91-17, 93-7, 93-8, 94-7, 94-18, 95-8, 95-26, 97-14, 98-10, 98-18, 98-21, 99-11, 99-14, 99-15, 99-29, 00-9, 00-16, 00-22, 00-34, 01-12, 02-14, 03-7, 03-22, 03-24, 04-1, 04-15, 05-9, 05-20
Chesterfield BP	80-13, 81-7
Chiles WD	69-6, 69-9, 69-10, 69-14, 69-16, 71-17, 71-28, 72-5, 72-11, 72-19, 72-21, 74-10, 75-10, 75-14, 76-1, 76-11, 77-15, 77-17, 78-19, 78-33, 78-34, 79-7
Chittum CB	89-14, 92-27, 95-22, 96-18, 98-2, 98-3, 99-10
Chubb GP	96-19, 97-6
Cierebiej A	69-18, 71-9
Clark G	66-5, 66-26, 66-34, 69-19
Clough DL	88-5
Cobb BB Jr	62-2, 62-3, 63-31, 65-19, 65-22, 67-1, 68-14, 71-30, 71-36, 71-40, 72-18, 72-22, 72-33, 73-7, 74-2, 74-7, 74-8, 75-3, 76-6
Coffey JD	96-12
Colangelo EJ	89-3
Collins WE	62-17, 63-3, 63-13, 63-14, 63-29, Tech. Pub.#1, 64-14, 64-15, 64-16, 65-1, 65-2, 65-17, 65-18, 65-24, 66-37, 67-2, 67-6, 67-7, 67-12, 67-19, 68-2, 68-10, 68-28, 69-15, 69-20, 70-10, 70-17, 71-20, 71-30, 71-31, 71-34, 71-39, 72-34, 72-35, 73-17, 73-18, 74-2, 74-3, 74-7, 75-1, 75-3, 75-4, 76-12, 76-14, 77-24, 78-13, 79-7, 79-9, 79-26, 80-7, 81-15, 81-16, 82-19, 83-6, 84-6, 85-3, 85-5, 86-9, 87-4, 88-2, 88-3, 89-7, 90-1, 90-4, 91-8, 92-1, 93-2, 94-1, 95-1, 95-3, 95-7, 95-13, 96-1, 96-21, 96-22, 97-1, 98-1, 99-1, 00-1, 01-1, 03-1, 05-1, 05-3
Coltman JW	83-3
Comerford DA	02-3, 03-5
Comperatore C	00-10
Connor CW	03-12, 04-9
Constant GN	73-19, 76-4
Convey JJ	83-11, 85-7, 86-6
Cook EA	72-30, 78-23
Copeland K	00-5, 03-16, 05-14
Corbett CL	01-18, 02-16, 03-15, 04-2, 04-12, 05-2
Cosper DK	98-1, 04-19
Court MC	97-20
Craft KJ	05-20
Crain RA	65-17, 66-2
Crane CR	63-27, 67-21, 70-4, 70-13, 72-12, 77-9, 78-26, 83-12, 85-4, 86-1, 86-3, 86-5, 86-8, 89-4, 90-15
Cremer RL	84-1
Crosby WM	68-6, 68-24, 69-3, 69-5
Crutchfield J	99-3
Cruz CE	95-12, 95-19, 96-23, 00-10, 02-8, 02-13, 02-20, 04-22, 04-23, 05-13, 06-13
Culver JF	62-12

D

Author	Report Number
Dailey JT	77-25, 78-35, 82-11, 84-2
Darden EB Jr	78-8
Dark SJ	76-10, 78-25, 80-19, 83-5, 84-9, 85-9, 86-7, 90-5
Dattel AR	06-16
Daugherty JW	62-10, 63-4
Davis AW Jr	63-12, 68-15, 68-18, 70-8, 77-17, 78-20, 78-25, 80-8, 84-4, 85-12, 90-7
Davis HV	71-41
Davis J	06-1
Dean MA	00-15
Deimler JD	94-21, 94-22, 94-23

DeJohn CA ------- 97-2, 97-21, 00-13, 04-16
Delafield RH ----- 69-12
Della Rocco PS--- 89-6, 90-13, 92-30, 95-12, 95-19, 96-23, 99-2, 00-10, 00-32
Deloney JR ------- 83-7
deSteiguer D ------ 78-4, 80-18, 83-10, 83-14
Detwiler C -------- 02-8, 02-13, 02-20, 02-24, 03-20, 03-11, 05-24, 06-7, 06-18
DeWeese R -------- 92-20, 93-14, 94-19, 95-30, 98-11, 02-11, 03-9, 04-18
Diehl AE ---------- 87-6
Dill DB ------------ 63-33
Dillard A ---------- 03-12, 04-9
Dille JR ----------- 62-12, 63-2, 63-21, 63-24, 63-27, 66-14, 66-27, 68-8, 68-16, 72-1, 74-1, 76-7, 77-1, 77-20, 79-19, 80-11, 81-1, 81-14, 83-1, 83-18, 84-7, 87-1
Dillon RD --------- 81-7
Dittmar MJ ------- 97-3
Dobbins L --------- 06-26
Dodd RS ---------- 96-3
Dollar CS --------- 87-4, 90-8, 94-13, 96-21, 97-17, 02-9, 03-14, 04-21, 06-30
Domino D -------- 03-2
Donnelly SS ------ 00-6
Dougherty MRP - 97-22, 98-16, 01-16, 02-1, 02-22
Downey LE ------- 90-5
Drechsler GK ----- 93-1, 95-16
Drilling HS ------- 03-23
Driskill WE ------- 97-3, 97-23, 98-7
Druray CG -------- 91-16
Dubowski KM --- 04-13, 05-9
Duke F ------------ 00-33
Duncan JC -------- 63-30
Durso FT --------- 98-26, 99-3, 00-5, 01-16

E

Eanuel TW Jr ----- 03-3
Earley JC ---------- 62-7
Eddington DL ---- 06-10
Edwards MB ------ 92-31, 94-3, 95-4, 95-9
Elam GW --------- 73-17, 81-16, 82-19
Emanuel T -------- 97-11
Emerson TE Jr --- 62-18, 63-1, 63-16, 63-22, 66-11
Endecott BR ------ 70-3, 77-9, 77-19, 83-12, 85-4 86-1 86-3 86-5 89-4, 90-15, 90-16, 91-17, 93-7, 93-8, 94-7, 94-18, 00-21
Endsley MR ------ 94-27, 97-13

England HM ----- 89-10, 92-18, 92-22, 93-6, 94-10
Enos RJ ------------ 99-24
Ericson SC -------- 04-7, 06-27

F

Faaborg T --------- 05-24
Fairlie GW -------- 91-6, 92-27
Farmer WL -------- 96-13, 97-4, 98-24, 99-16, 00-3, 01-4
Faulkner DN ----- 78-8, 82-12, 92-2
Feinberg R -------- 65-9, 65-25
Ferrante A --------- 03-19
Ferraro DP -------- 73-12, 75-6
Fiedler ER --------- 00-32, 01-11, 02-23
Fineg J ------------- 68-24
Fiorica V ---------- 66-6, 66-11, 66-14, 66-41, 68-4, 68-15, 68-23, 70-8, 70-18 71-11 71-15 71-23 71-41
Fisher RG --------- 74-4
Flemig JW -------- 94-14, 95-28
Flux M ------------- 77-3, 77-16, 82-5
Folk ED ----------- 70-18, 72-30, 73-10, 82-8, 92-27
Forster EM -------- 06-5
Fotouhi CH ------ 96-6
Fowler PR --------- 63-8, 67-5, 75-7, 77-17, 80-10, 83-2
Fox CM ----------- 01-10, 02-4
Freud SL ---------- 64-9, 64-10, 64-17, 66-25
Friedberg W ------ 71-26, 78-8, 80-2, 82-12, 92-2, 00-33, 03-16, 05-14
Fromhagen C ----- 71-18
Fulk GW ---------- 91-1
Fuller DK --------- 94-3, 95-4
Funkhouser GE -- 63-25, 66-14, 67-4, 67-17, 68-13, 68-15, 68-18, 70-5, 71-2, 71-17, 72-17, 73-22, 75-10, 75-14, 76-11, 77-8, 77-17, 78-19, 79-10, 80-10, 81-8, 82-10, 83-2, 83-14, 85-10, 87-2, 89-8, 89-11, 91-6, 92-27, 95-20, 95-22, 96-18, 98-3, 99-10

G

Galaxy SciCorp --- 93-5, 93-15, 94-12, 95-14, 96-2
Galerston EM ---- 68-13, 68-18
Ganslen RV ------- 63-12, 63-34
Garber M --------- 00-29, 01-12
Garner JD --------- 62-1, 62-9, 65-7, 66-42, 70-19, 72-30, 77-11, 78-3, 78-23, 79-22, 80-12
Garner RP -------- 94-10, 95-17, 95-29, 96-4, 97-7, 98-4, 98-27, 99-4, 00-6, 04-3, 04-7, 05-18, 06-10, 06-27
Gay DJ ------------ 77-24
Geiwitz KL -------- 00-6

Part II: Author Index

Author	Report Number	Author	Report Number
George MH	91-2, 91-3, 95-20, 95-22, 95-25, 96-18, 98-3, 99-5, 99-10	Hastings J	06-1
Gerathewohl SJ	69-17, 69-24, 70-9, 71-10, 71-33, 75-5, 77-6, 78-16, 78-27	Hattrup RA	05-11
		Hau G	06-10
Gerke RJ	72-4	Hauty GT	65-5, 65-6, 65-16, 65-28, 65-29, 65-30
Gibbons HL	68-8, 69-9, 69-10, 71-18	Hawkes GR	62-11, 62-16
Gilcher RO	84-4	Heil MC	99-18, 99-23, 00-12, 01-5, 01-4, 01-6, 02-24
Giles E	79-2		
Gilliland K	93-13, 97-5, 97-25, 99-20	Heil SKR	01-4
Gilson RD	71-20, 71-34, 72-34	Hellman CM	91-15, 92-13, 93-18
Gogel WC	62-15, 63-10, 63-20, 63-28, 64-13, 65-11, 65-32, 66-22, 66-24, 67-18, 67-20	Hendrix AM	03-13, 95-15, 06-25
		Hendrix R	06-25
Goldman RF	62-5	Higgins EA	63-23, 66-14, 66-39, 68-13, 68-15, 68-18, 69-10, 70-5, 70-8, 71-17, 71-41, 72-17, 73-22, 75-10, 75-14, 76-11, 77-8, 77-17, 78-5, 78-19, 79-10, 79-20, 80-9, 80-10, 81-8, 82-10, 83-2, 83-4, 83-14, 85-5, 85-10, 85-11, 87-2, 87-5, 89-5, 89-8, 89-10, 89-11, 89-12
Goldman SM	02-23, 04-22, 04-23, 06-4, 06-26		
Good GW	05-21		
Goulden DR	71-5, 72-16, 73-19, 76-4, 81-4, 83-17		
Gowdy RV	90-11, 92-20, 93-14, 94-19, 98-11, 99-5, 02-11, 03-9		
		Hill RJ	71-39
Grape PM	77-8, 78-13, 80-3, 81-15, 82-15, 85-8	Hill TJ	93-19
Grimm EJ	72-16, 73-19, 75-4, 76-4	Hillman DJ	94-22
Grimm MH	72-1, 74-1, 87-1	Hilton Systems Inc	94-20
Gronlund SD	97-22, 98-16, 01-16, 02-1, 02-22	Hilton TF	97-8, 97-12, 99-19, 00-3
Guedry FE Jr	67-6, 67-7, 71-20, 71-34, 72-34	Hinshaw LB	62-18, 63-1, 63-16, 63-22, 63-26, 63-32, 66-11
Guilkey JE	98-6		
Gurman EB	94-21	Hodges BE	03-10
		Hoffman SM	69-12, 72-17, 73-21, 73-22, 74-11, 75-7, 76-13, 77-5

H

Hackworth CA	98-26, 99-3, 03-10, 03-11, 04-22, 04-23, 05-13, 06-7, 06-13, 06-18	Holcomb K	02-20, 05-24, 06-7 06-18
		Holland J	02-21
Hand DK	97-3, 97-23, 98-7	Holloway FA	94-24
Hanneman GD	70-3, 77-8, 78-8, 81-11, 84-5, 87-3, 87-8	Holmes DD	63-23, 63-26, 66-11
Hanson PG	68-6, 68-24, 69-5, 69-13	Hordinsky JR	91-2, 91-3, 92-11, 92-19, 92-23, 94-14, 94-16, 95-28, 97-2, 98-10, 00-21
Hansrote RW	97-21		
Haraway A	81-1, 83-1	Houk VN	64-7
Harper CR	66-30	Houston ER	98-5
Harris HC Jr	95-3, 95-7, 96-16, 97-24, 99-22, 05-7, 05-12	Hudgins CB	98-4, 98-27
		Hudson LS	90-7
Harris JL	84-7	Huffine EF	92-24, 92-25, 99-15
Harris RM	94-22	Huffman HW	64-15
Harrison HF	66-16, 70-21	Hufnagel CA	64-7
Hart IS	00-3	Huggins ME	04-1, 06-14
Hartel CEJ	95-21	Hulin CL	97-11, 03-3
Hartel GF	95-21	Hunter CE	65-31
Hartman S	79-2	Hunter DR	95-27, 96-19, 97-3, 97-6, 97-16, 97-23, 98-6, 98-7, 99-7, 02-17
Hasbrook AH	62-7, 62-9, 62-13, 65-14, 66-32, 68-12, 68-22, 70-7, 71-24, 72-9, 72-27, 73-9, 73-23, 75-12, 77-24		
		Huntley MS Jr	91-7, 91-13
		Hurst MW	78-39
		Hutto GL	72-24, 77-21, 81-5
		Hyde AS	63-30

Author	Report Number	Author	Report Number
Hyland DT	94-21, 94-22, 94-23	Kirkbride LA	96-19
Hynes MK	99-30, 00-11	Kirkham WR	78-13, 80-3, 80-6, 81-10, 81-15, 82-7, 82-13, 83-8

I

Iampietro PF	62-5, 62-18, 63-1, 63-23, 66-14, 66-23, 68-15, 69-10, 70-8, 70-22, 71-2, 71-4, 71-17, 72-17, 72-35, 75-10, 75-14	Knecht W	02-20, 05-7, 05-15
		Knowlan DM	64-11
		Kochan JA	97-6
Ice J	63-30	Korty P	62-10, 63-4
Irons FM	73-13, 73-20	Kot PA	64-11
Isaac A	02-12, 03-21	Kranz G	70-10
		Kupfer DM	00-16, 06-14
		Kupiec TC	92-24, 96-14, 96-17, 97-14

J

L

Jack DG	03-10, 04-22, 04-23, 05-13, 06-20		
Jahns DW	99-9, 00-4	Lacefield DJ	78-31, 82-15, 85-8
Jeffress LA	63-7	Lacey DE	62-10, 63-4
Jenkins CD	78-39	Lacy CD	71-5
Jennings AE	69-10, 69-14, 72-5, 72-11, 72-21, 75-10, 75-14, 76-1, 76-11, 77-17, 78-19, 78-33, 78-34, 78-37	LaJonchere CM	99-28
		Lamb MW	96-3
		Lambrou P	99-22
Jennings R	06-1	Lamonica J	00-26
Jensen RS	96-19, 97-6, 98-6, 99-7	Langston ED	72-6, 72-7
Johansson J	02-1, 02-22	Larcher JG	00-13, 02-16, 04-12, 04-16
Johnson RD	00-20, 02-15, 03-18, 03-23, 04-4, 04-13, 05-10, 05-11, 06-3, 06-5, 06-17, 06-19	Lategola MT	63-11, 66-16, 66-17, 66-20, 66-21, 70-8, 70-18, 70-21, 71-8, 71-19, 72-20, 72-26, 73-10, 74-6, 77-3, 77-16, 78-5, 78-20, 79-8, 79-20, 80-9, 81-2, 82-3, 82-4, 82-5, 84-4
Johnson WB	91-16		
Jones D	06-1		
Jones JP	92-31	Lay CD	71-36, 72-22
Jones KN	71-5, 71-7, 71-29, 72-14, 72-16, 72-25, 73-14, 75-1	Layne PJ	74-6
		Layton CF	95-31
Jordan JL	82-14, 06-1	Leeper RC	73-23
Josenhans WKT	65-8	Lendrum L	03-3
Joseph KM	99-9, 99-17, 99-25, 99-27, 00-4, 00-14, 03-2	Lennon AO	75-4, 77-24
		Lentz JM	76-14

K

		Lester LF	87-6
		Leverett S Jr	63-30
Kanki BG	96-10	Lewis MA	78-7, 78-36, 79-3, 79-14
Karim B	72-27	Lewis MF	67-8, 67-16, 67-24, 68-20, 68-27, 70-15, 71-27, 71-32, 71-42, 72-29, 73-6, 73-12, 73-18, 75-6, 79-4, 81-6, 82-6
Karson S	70-14		
Kay EJ	94-21, 94-22, 94-23		
Keen FR	66-31	Lewis RA	69-6, 69-16
Kegg PS	88-3	Lewis RJ	99-15, 00-20, 00-29, 02-15, 03-18, 03-23, 04-4, 04-13, 04-15, 05-8, 05-10, 05-11, 06-3, 06-5, 06-12, 06-17, 06-19
Kendall WW	63-25		
Key OR	97-21		
Kidd GD Jr	79-5	Li G	96-3
King RE	02-23, 02-24, 03-20, 06-16	Lieberman P	98-20
King SJ	03-11, 04-22, 04-23, 05-13	Linder MK	80-11
Kinn JB	68-3	Lintern G	97-11
		Lia TL	05-8

Part II: Author Index

Author	Report Number
Liu RH	05-8
Loewenfeld I	65-9
Lofberg MS	83-16
Loochan FK	91-14, 92-14
Lowenstein O	65-9
Lowrey DL	72-6, 77-11, 78-3, 79-22, 80-12, 80-13, 82-7, 82-13, 83-8
Luchsinger PC	64-8
Lyne PJ	63-8, 73-10, 77-3, 77-16, 78-20, 81-2, 82-3, 82-4, 84-4, 85-10, 87-2, 89-8, 89-10, 89-11, 89-12
Lynn CA	73-10

M

Author	Report Number
Maclin O	96-20
Madakasira S	92-11
Mandella JG Jr	95-29, 98-4, 98-27, 05-18
Manning CA	84-6, 88-3, 89-6, 90-4, 90-6, 90-13, 91-9, 92-5, 92-26, 92-31, 94-3, 94-9, 95-4, 95-9, 96-5 97-15, 97-22, 98-16, 98-26, 99-3, 00-2, 00-5, 01-5, 01-6, 01-10, 02-2, 02-4, 05-4, 06-4, 06-21, 06-29
Marcus JH	93-14, 94-11, 96-7, 96-11, 97-18, 97-20
Marsh DK II	98-9
Mastrullo AR	81-15
Masucci FD	63-22
Mathews JJ	72-18, 72-22, 72-33, 73-7, 74-2, 74-7, 75-3
May ND	92-4
McCauley ME	01-17
McClenathan JE	64-7
McConville JT	76-9
McCoy J	66-17
McDown JR	02-16, 04-12
McFadden EB	62-13, 62-21, 63-9, 65-7, 66-7, 66-13, 66-20, 67-3, 67-4, 67-9, 70-20, 71-37, 72-10, 78-1, 78-4, 78-9, 79-13
McKenzie JM	63-8, 66-41, 67-5, 71-2, 71-21, 73-21, 73-22, 74-11, 75-7, 75-10, 75-14, 76-11, 76-13, 76-15, 77-17, 77-23, 78-18, 78-19, 78-30, 78-40, 79-10, 79-20, 80-10, 81-8, 81-13, 82-10, 83-2, 83-4
McLean GA	89-8, 89-10, 89-11, 89-12, 91-12, 92-18, 92-22, 92-27, 93-6, 93-19, 95-22, 95-25, 96-18, 98-2, 98-3, 98-19, 99-5, 99-10, 01-2, 02-16, 03-15, 04-2, 04-12, 04-19
McLin L	03-12, 04-9
Mehling KD	71-31
Mejdal S	01-17

Author	Report Number
Melton CE Jr	63-5, 64-18, 66-35, 66-39, 67-15, 68-26, 69-1, 69-12, 71-2, 71-21, 71-23, 72-17, 73-15, 73-21, 73-22, 74-11, 75-7, 76-2, 76-13, 77-5, 77-23, 78-5, 78-18, 78-40, 79-20, 80-9, 80-16, 81-13, 82-17, 85-2, 86-2, 89-13
Melton RJ	79-23
Mertens HW	65-32, 66-22, 66-38, 67-20, 67-24, 68-27, 70-15, 71-42, 72-29, 75-6, 77-12, 78-15, 79-4, 79-25, 81-6, 81-8, 82-6, 82-10, 83-4, 83-15, 85-3, 85-5, 88-2, 90-9, 92-6, 92-28, 92-29, 92-30, 93-16, 93-17, 95-13, 96-22, 97-10, 99-8, 04-14
Mertens RA	67-2, 68-7, 70-10, 71-5
Mielnik T	06-10
Milburn NJ	82-10, 92-28, 92-29, 92-30, 93-16, 93-17, 95-13, 96-22, 97-10, 99-8, 04-10, 04-14, 06-26
Milke RM	99-22
Millett DP	00-21
Mills SH	97-7, 98-15, 00-30, 01-10, 01-16, 02-1, 02-2, 02-4, 02-22
Mills W	01-11
Moertl PM	00-5, 02-1, 02-22
Mogford LS	98-14
Mogford RH	98-14
Mogilka HJ	01-10, 02-4
Mohler SR	62-4, 62-20, 63-2, 65-7, 65-13, 66-1, 66-3, 66-8, 66-25, 66-29, 66-30, 66-31, 66-32, 67-22, 68-8, 68-16, 69-2, 69-17, 69-18, 70-12, 71-9, 71-10, 71-33, 72-2, 72-28, 75-5, 80-4, 96-25, 06-1
Moise S	92-11
Montgomery RW	93-21, 94-15, 95-11, 96-12, 99-6, 00-19, 00-23, 01-7, 01-14, 02-6, 02-10, 03-6, 03-12, 04-6, 04-9, 05-21, 06-9, 06-23, 06-28
Moorcroft D	04-18
Moore CM	69-19
Morgan JC	68-26
Morris Edward W	66-27
Morris Everett W	70-9
Morrison JE	96-6
Morrow DG	99-21
Moser E	83-2
Moser KM	64-5, 64-7, 64-8
Moses R	66-14, 68-4, 71-11, 71-15, 80-10
Mullen SR	77-17, 78-19, 79-10
Murcko LE	76-4, 77-1
Murphy RE	98-4, 98-27, 00-6
Myers JG	90-2, 91-5, 91-10, 92-15, 92-16, 95-10

N

Naff KC ---------- 00-27
Nagle FJ ---------- 63-12, 63-34, 64-2, 66-36
Nakagawara VB -- 90-10, 91-1, 91-14, 92-14, 93-11, 93-21, 94-10, 94-15, 95-11, 96-12, 96-27, 98-25, 99-6, 00-18, 00-19, 00-23, 01-7, 01-14, 02-6, 02-10, 03-6, 03-12, 04-6, 04-9, 05-21, 06-9, 06-23, 06-28
Nance C ---------- 00-26
Naughton J -------- 64-2, 66-17, 66-21, 66-36
Neal GL ---------- 65-31
Neas BR ---------- 78-8, 80-2
Neddick M -------- 99-9
Nelson JM -------- 71-26
Nelson PL --------- 72-33, 73-7, 74-8
Nesthus TE ------- 95-5, 95-7, 97-7, 97-9, 97-25, 99-20, 02-8, 02-13, 02-20, 06-13
Newton JL -------- 63-33
Newton NL ------- 62-12
Nguyen K --------- 0032
Nicholas J --------- 00-33
Nichols EA -------- 72-2
Nikolic D --------- 99-3
Norwood GK ----- 71-25, 71-38, 82-14
Nye LG ----------- 89-7, 90-4, 90-8, 91-8, 92-7, 92-8, 92-9, 92-10, 94-13

O

O'Brien K --------- 00-33
O'Connor WF --- 65-10, 66-10, 66-15
O'Dell JW -------- 70-14
O'Doherty DS --- 65-4
Odom RS --------- 02-16
O'Donnell RD --- 92-11, 95-24
Ohrt DD ---------- 97-22, 98-16
Olmos BO -------- 03-2
Orme DR --------- 01-11
Orzechowski JA -- 04-7, 06-27
OU Vortac -------- 92-31, 94-3, 95-4, 95-9, 96-5
Owuor ED -------- 04-1
Ozur H ------------ 82-11

P

Packingham KD - 99-28
Page BB ----------- 63-22
Palmerton DA ---- 98-3, 98-13, 02-16, 04-12, 05-17
Parker JF Jr ------- 89-9, 90-14, 95-2
Patterson JC ------ 01-11
Pearson DW ------ 68-17, 69-7, 69-19
Pearson RG ------- 63-35, 65-10, 65-31, 66-19
Pendergrass GE --- 63-27, 66-10, 66-15
Penland T --------- 85-1
Pennybaker AL --- 96-25
Perloff JK --------- 64-19
Perry JL ----------- 98-16
Perry RB ----------- 64-8
Peterson LM ------ 00-28, 01-19, 01-20, 03-10
Pfleiderer EM ----- 00-24, 01-10, 02-2, 02-4, 03-8, 05-16, 06-4, 06-7, 06-29
Phillips EE -------- 63-34
Phillips S ---------- 97-11
Pickett E ----------- 98-20
Pickrel EW -------- 77-25, 79-18, 82-11, 83-11, 84-2
Pidkowicz JK ----- 80-8
Pinkerson AL ----- 64-11
Pinski MS --------- 78-4, 78-14
Podolak E --------- 65-25, 68-3
Polis BD ----------- 71-2, 73-21, 73-22
Pollard DW ------- 78-3, 79-6, 79-23, 82-8, 84-1, 85-1
Porter KA --------- 02-16
Pounds J ----------- 99-12, 02-12, 03-19, 03-21, 05-5, 05-25, 06-20, 06-21, 06-26
Price GT ---------- 69-3, 69-13, 74-4, 77-8
Prinzo OV -------- 93-20, 95-15, 96-10, 96-20, 96-26, 98-17, 98-20, 99-21, 01-8, 01-9, 02-5, 03-13, 04-11, 05-19, 06-25
Purswell JL -------- 72-27, 73-23

Q

Quebe J ------------ 97-3, 98-7

R

Raeke JW --------- 62-21
Ramos RA --------- 01-5, 01-6
Rana B ------------- 75-9
Rantanen E ------- 03-3
Rasmussen PG --- 70-7, 71-24, 72-9, 73-9, 75-12, 77-2, 77-7, 77-13, 77-14, 78-17, 78-22, 78-28, 78-29, 78-41, 79-22, 80-13, 81-7, 89-14, 92-12, 94-8
Reed W ------------ 72-6, 73-1
Reighard HL ------ 65-3, 76-8, 78-35
Reins DA ---------- 63-26, 65-27, 66-11
Retzlaff PD -------- 03-20

Part II: Author Index

Author	Report Number
Revzin AM	70-11, 73-3, 73-4, 77-22, 78-2, 79-15, 92-12, 94-8
Reynolds HI	67-4
Reynolds HM	75-2, 75-13, 76-9, 82-9
Rice N	70-10
Rieger JA Jr	66-11
Ritter RM	93-7, 93-8, 94-7, 98-18, 98-21, 03-23
Rizutti BL	76-6
Roberts PA	78-31, 82-15, 85-8
Robinette KM	83-16
Robinson CP	77-19, 78-26
Robinson S	63-33
Rock DB	82-11
Rodgers MD	93-1, 93-9, 93-12, 93-22, 94-27, 95-16, 95-18, 97-13, 98-14, 06-20
Roe BA	00-16
Rohrbaugh JW	99-28
Rosa RR	95-32
Rose RM	78-39
Ross A	67-22
Rotter AJ	92-31
Rowlan DE	72-15
Rowland RC Jr	67-10
Roy KM	02-19
Rubenstein CJ	93-19
Ruehle C	06-1
Rueschhoff BJ	85-11
Rush L	97-9
Russell CJ	00-15
Russell JC	85-12, 89-3
Ryan LC	70-3, 75-5, 80-4
Rylander R	73-11

S

Author	Report Number
Sahiar F	96-25
Salazar GJ	97-21, 06-1, 06-12
Saldivar JT	66-39, 68-26, 72-17, 73-21, 73-22, 74-11, 75-7, 76-13, 77-5, 77-23, 78-18, 78-40, 80-18, 81-13 83-10, 83-14, 85-10, 87-2
Sanders DC	67-21, 70-4, 70-13, 72-12, 77-9, 83-12, 85-4, 86-1, 86-3, 86-5, 86-8, 89-4, 90-15, 90-16, 91-17, 93-7, 93-8, 94-7, 94-18, 95-8, 98-10
Sangal SP	95-5
Sauer HH	05-14
Scarborough A	05-25
Scarborough WR	64-12, 65-8, 65-15
Scarpa P	06-1
Schlegel RE	93-13, 97-5, 97-25, 98-13, 99-20
Schlegel TT	89-10
Schroeder DJ	68-10, 70-10, 71-6, 71-16, 71-20, 71-31, 71-34, 71-39, 72-34, 73-17, 79-9, 81-16, 82-19, 83-7, 83-17, 87-4, 89-7, 90-6, 90-8, 92-7, 93-4, 94-6, 94-13, 94-17, 94-26, 95-3, 95-7, 95-32, 96-9, 97-17, 99-17, 99-22, 00-32, 03-14, 03-20, 04-21, 05-5, 05-22, 06-2, 06-6, 06-21
Schvaneveldt R	00-26
Scow J	66-15
Seipel JH	64-6, 65-4, 67-11
Sells SB	84-2
Sershon JL	84-5, 87-3, 87-8
Shaftstall RM	02-16, 06-10, 06-19
Shanbour K	66-17, 66-21
Shappell SA	00-7, 01-3, 03-4, 05-7, 05-24, 06-7, 06-18, 06-24
Shaw RV	96-24
Shehab RL	98-13
Shepherd WT	89-9, 90-14, 91-16, 95-2, 95-14, 95-31, 96-2
Siegel PV	67-25, 68-9, 69-2, 69-17, 69-18, 71-10
Silberman WS	06-1
Simcox LS	84-3
Simpson JM	66-13, 67-9, 78-13, 80-3
Simpson LP	81-4
Sirevaag EJ	99-28
Sirkis JA	70-9, 72-3
Smith DR	00-9, 00-21, 02-14, 00-34
Smith LT	93-19
Smith MD	98-5, 98-21
Smith PW	62-8, 63-24, 69-9, 70-3, 77-9, 77-19, 78-26
Smith RC	70-20, 71-14, 71-21, 71-28, 71-30, 71-35, 72-23, 72-24, 73-2, 73-15, 73-22, 74-12, 75-7, 75-9, 76-2, 76-13, 77-21, 77-23, 78-32, 79-11, 80-14, 81-5
Snow CC	62-9, 65-14, 65-26, 68-6, 68-19, 68-24, 69-3, 69-4, 69-5, 69-13, 70-16, 72-27, 75-2, 79-2, 82-9
Snyder L	77-8, 82-12, 92-2
Snyder RG	62-13, 62-19, 63-15, 63-30, 65-12, 65-26, 68-6, 68-19, 68-24, 69-3, 69-4, 69-5, 69-13, 76-9
Solomon LA	66-11
Soper JW	96-17, 99-29, 00-16, 02-14, 03-22, 03-24
Southern TL	00-29
Spera S	06-10
Spieth W	64-4

Author	Report Number
St George R	99-9
Staggs CM	85-6
Stavinoha WB	66-11
Stedman VG	71-9
Steen JA	71-27, 71-32, 72-29, 73-18, 75-1, 75-6, 80-5, 80-15, 84-1, 85-1
Stern JA	94-6, 94-17, 94-26, 96-9, 99-28
Stoliarov N	94-6, 94-26, 96-9
Stutzman TM	91-5
Swearingen JJ	62-1, 62-4, 62-13, 62-14, 63-9, 65-7, 65-20, 65-23, 66-3, 66-12, 66-18, 66-40, 67-14, 69-22, 71-3, 71-12, 71-13, 72-6, 72-7, 72-15, 73-1

T

Author	Report Number
Taite S	05-23
Talleur DA	97-11, 03-3
Tang PC	63-21
Taylor DK	75-9, 81-15, 83-6, 84-6
Taylor HL	97-11, 03-3
Taylor JC	91-16
Teague SM	92-19
Thackray RI	68-17, 69-7, 69-8, 69-21, 71-7, 71-29, 72-14, 72-25, 73-11, 73-14, 73-16, 74-9, 75-8, 77-18, 78-11, 79-12, 79-24, 80-1, 80-17, 81-5, 81-12, 82-1, 82-16, 83-13, 85-13, 86-4, 88-1, 88-4, 89-1, 90-3, 92-3, 92-6, 94-6
Thomas AA	71-41
Thomas JA	06-10
Thomas S	05-8
Thompson D	06-20
Thompson JJ	00-3
Thompson KE	00-6
Thompson RC	97-8, 97-12, 98-8, 98-24, 99-17, 99-19, 99-24, 99-25, 99-27, 00-14, 00-17, 00-25, 00-27, 00-28, 01-4
Thomson GL	97-22
Tilton FE	06-1
Tobias JV	63-7, 63-17, 63-19, Tech. Pub.#1, 64-16, 65-17, 66-4, 67-10, 68-21, 68-25, 70-6, 71-1, 72-31, 72-32, 73-13, 73-20, 75-11, 76-3, 79-5, 79-16
Touchstone RM	69-21, 71-29, 72-14, 72-25, 73-11, 73-14, 73-16, 74-9, 75-8, 77-18, 78-11, 79-12, 79-24, 80-17, 81-12, 82-1, 82-16, 83-13, 85-13, 86-4, 88-1, 89-1, 90-3, 92-6, 94-6, 94-26, 96-9
Trent CC	79-8
Trites DK	61-1, 62-3, 63-31, 65-5, 65-6, 65-21, 65-22
Trout EM	78-6, 78-12, 78-24, 79-17

Author	Report Number
Truitt TR	96-5, 98-26, 99-3, 00-5
Tucker R	00-26
Turner JW	91-7, 91-13
Twohig P	04-22
Tyler RR	02-21

U

Author	Report Number
Uhlarik J	02-3, 03-5
Umberger EL	66-25
Updegraff BP	69-20
Ultrecht JS	04-3

V

Author	Report Number
Valdez CD	77-4, 90-12
van Brummelen AG	65-8
VanBuskirk LK	80-5, 80-15
Vance FP	68-26
VanDeventer AD	80-7, 83-6, 84-6
Vant JHB	89-5
Vardaman JJ	94-5
Vaughan JA	68-13, 68-15, 68-18, 69-10, 70-5, 71-17, 72-17, 75-10, 75-14, 76-5, 76-11, 77-2, 77-7, 77-13, 77-14, 78-17, 78-22, 78-28, 78-29, 78-41, 79-20, 80-9
Vedeniapin AB	99-28
Veregge JE	66-25, 67-22, 67-23
Veronneau SJH	94-14, 95-5, 96-25, 97-2, 00-13, 00-18, 00-22
Ververs PM	98-28
Von Rosenberg CW	66-31
Voros RS	94-22
Vu NT	94-7, 98-18, 99-14, 00-16, 04-1, 04-4, 06-14

W

Author	Report Number
Wade K	01-15, 05-1, 05-3
Wallace TF	69-22, 72-15, 78-13, 80-3
Wang SM	05-8
Warner D	92-11
Wayda ME	90-1, 92-1, 94-1, 96-1, 97-1, 98-1, 99-1, 00-1, 01-1, 03-1, 05-1
Weigmann DA	00-7, 05-24, 06-7, 06-18, 06-24
Weissmuller JJ	97-3, 97-23, 98-7
Welsh KW	76-5, 77-2, 77-7, 77-13, 77-14 78-17 78-22 78-28 78-29 78-41
Wentz AE	64-1, 64-6
Wernick JS	63-19

Author Index

Author	Report Number
West G	71-17, 72-5, 72-19, 72-21, 74-10, 75-14
West RW	91-1
Westura EE	68-3
Wheelright CD	62-1
Whinnery JE	03-15, 04-1, 05-20, 06-1, 06-5, 06-12
White MA	83-2
White ME	82-10
White VL	92-23, 94-16, 96-14, 96-17, 00-22, 01-12, 04-1
Wick RL Jr	72-4
Wickens CD	98-28
Wicks SM	66-35, 66-39, 67-15, 68-26, 69-1, 77-23, 78-18, 78-40, 80-10, 81-13, 82-7, 82-13, 83-8
Wiegmann DA	01-3, 03-4, 05-24, 06-7, 06-18, 06-24
Wilcox BC Jr	91-12, 92-18, 92-22, 93-6, 94-10, 96-25
Willems BF	01-20, 02-18
Williams CA	00-14, 03-10, 03-17, 04-20
Williams CA	02-24
Williams KW	94-25, 95-6, 96-8, 98-12, 99-13, 99-26, 00-8, 00-28, 00-31, 01-13, 02-21, 04-20, 04-24, 06-8
Williams MJ	69-15
Williams SD	03-23
Willis DM	75-12
Wing H	91-9
Winget CM	75-10
Wise RA	97-7
Witt LA	91-10, 91-11, 91-15, 92-7, 92-8, 92-9, 92-10, 92-13, 92-17, 92-21, 93-18, 94-2, 95-32, 97-8
Wittmers LE	65-27
Wolbrink AM	04-16, 00-13
Wolf MB	98-4
Wong KL	04-7, 06-27
Wood KJ	91-14, 92-14, 93-11, 93-21, 94-15, 95-11, 96-27, 98-25, 99-6, 00-19, 01-14, 02-6, 02-10, 03-6, 04-6, 06-9, 06-23, 06-28
Worley JA	99-17, 99-25, 99-27, 00-14
Wreggit S	97-9, 98-9

X

Author	Report Number
Xing J	04-17, 05-4, 06-2, 06-6, 06-11, 06-15, 06-22

Y

Author	Report Number
Yanowitch EA	73-5
Yanowitch RE	72-2, 73-5
Yost A	02-21
Young CL	76-6
Young FA	79-2
Young JW	62-21, 65-23, 66-9, 66-33, 67-13, 69-3, 69-4, 69-5, 69-13, 71-37, 74-4, 76-9, 78-14, 82-9, 83-16, 89-8, 89-11, 93-10
Young PE	68-11, 68-12
Young WC	93-4, 96-13, 97-4

Z

Author	Report Number
Zehner GF	83-16
Zeiner AR	72-8
Zelenski JD	77-19
Zhu H	04-1
Ziemnowicz SAR	65-4

PART III: SUBJECT INDEX

Subject and Report Number

Acceleration, angular

...adaptation, 66-37, 67-6, 67-7, 67-12, 67-19, 69-20, 74-3

...antimotion sickness drugs effects, 81-16, 82-19

...alcohol effects, 71-6, 71-16, 71-20, 71-34, 71-39, 72-34, 95-3

...arousal effects on nystagmus, 62-17

...arousal effects on vestibular response, 63-29

...dextroamphetamine effects on performance, 73-17, 76-12

...nystagmus after caloric habituation, 63-14, 64-14, 65-18, 67-2

...nystagmus after rotation habituation, 63-13, 65-24, 68-2

...rotation device, 64-15

...secobarbital effects on performance, 73-17

...sleep loss effects on performance, 76-12, 86-9

Acceleration, linear (see also Deceleration)

...bibliography, 63-30

Accidents

...age of pilots, 77-10, 04-8

...agricultural aircraft, 66-27, 66-30, 72-15, 78-31, 80-3

...Alaskan CFIT, evaluated by HFACS, 00-28, 06-7

...alcohol involved, 66-29, 68-16, 78-31, 80-4, 92-24, 98-5, 00-21, 03-18, 03-23, 04-13, 05-20

...analyses of injuries, 70-16, 71-3, 72-15, 81-10, 82-7, 05-17

...analytic methodology of causal factors, 06-26

...bloodborne pathogens, 97-21

...cabin injuries, 79-23, 82-8

...carbon monoxide levels without fire, 80-11, 00-18, 00-34, 05-9

...cocaine and associated metabolites, analytic method, 03-23, 03-24

...causes, 66-8, 66-27, 66-29, 67-23, 68-16, 69-2, 70-18, 78-13, 82-15, 05-9, 05-20, 05-24, 06-24

...cockpit delethalization, 66-3, 66-12, 71-3

...controlled flight into terrain, human error analysis, 03-4

...coronary atherosclerosis in pilot fatalities, 80-8, 85-6

...drugs and toxic chemicals as causes, 68-16, 78-31, 85-8, 95-28, 96-17, 00-9, 00-21, 00-29, 00-34, 03-7, 03-22, 03-23, 03-24, 05-20

...evacuation injuries, 79-6, 80-12, 99-30, 00-11

...evacuation patterns, 62-9, 65-7, 70-16, 96-18

...experience of pilots, 77-10

Subject and Report Number

...fatalities identification, 79-2, 98-18, 06-14

...fire, smoke protection, 67-4, 70-16, 70-20, 78-4, 83-10, 85-10

...glare involvement, 03-6, 06-28

...glucose levels, abnormal, 00-22

...HFACS, human factors analysis and classification system for human error, 00-7

   –applied to air carriers and commuter accidents, 06-18

   –applied to Alaskan CFIT accidents, 00-28

   –applied to general aviation CFIT accidents, 03-4

   –applied to general aviation accidents, 1990-2000, 05-24

   –applied to general aviation accidents in Alaska, 06-7

   –in conjunction with intervention programs, 06-24

...in-flight incapacitation, 87-7, 04-16

...in-flight vertigo and unconsciousness, 63-21

...injuries, from seat impacts, 66-18

   –in extreme vertical impacts, 62-19

   –in rearward-facing seats, 62-7

...instructional flights, 96-3

...intervention programs, 06-24

...investigations, human factors findings, 63-35, 69-18, 72-2, 73-5, 80-6, 04-24, 05-24, 06-24

...lapbelt-restraint injuries to pregnant females, 68-24

...lost/disoriented, 95-1

...occupation of pilots, 77-10

...older pilots, 67-22, 70-18, 04-8

...padding for crash protection, 66-40

...physician pilots, 66-25, 71-9

...pilots with static physical defects, 76-7, 77-20, 79-19, 81-14, 83-18, 93-11

...post mortem findings, 69-18, 92-23, 92-24, 92-25, 94-14, 95-28, 97-14, 98-18, 00-9, 00-16, 00-29, 03-4, 03-22, 03-24, 04-13, 05-9, 05-10, 05-11, 05-20, 06-3, 06-14, 06-17

   –in relation to medical history, 06-12

   –quality assurance of forensic analyses, 99-11, 99-14, 99-15, 99-29, 03-18, 04-1, 04-4, 04-13, 04-15, 06-14

...predisposition, 72-2, 73-5, 93-9

...prevention with blind flight instrument, 66-32

...propeller-to-person, 81-15, 93-2

...railroad, 73-1

...risk factors, for controlled flight into terrain (Alaska), 00-28

   –for marginal weather take-offs by general aviation pilots, 05-7, 05-15

...rotorcraft, rollover and injury/fatality rates, 05-17
...safety information for improved survival, 04-19
...seat cushions for flotation, 66-13, 98-19
...shoulder harnesses to increase survival, 72-3, 83-8, 89-3
...spatial disorientation, 78-13, 95-1, 96-21
...stall warning, 66-31
...suicide, 72-2, 73-5, 06-5
...survivability, fire/smoke, 95-8, 05-17
 –free-fall impacts, 63-15
 –water impacts, 65-12, 68-19
...triamterene in blood, identification of, 92-23
...unmanned aircraft, accidents and incidents, 04-24
 –flight-control problems, 06-8
...visual acuity of pilots, 75-5, 81-14, 83-18, 00-18
...water spray systems, 98-4
...water survival, analysis of training programs, 98-19
 –frequency of occurrence, 98-19
...WinMine analytic tool applied to accident data, 06-26

Aerial application

...accidents, 66-27, 66-30, 68-16, 72-15, 78-31, 80-3
...biochemical effects of lindane and dieldrin, 62-10, 63-4
...chlordimeform toxicity, 77-19
...cholinesterase determination, 67-5
...comparison of serum cholinesterase methods, 70-13, 72-12
...dieldrin effects on liver, 66-5, 66-26
...endrin effects, 66-11, 66-26, 66-34, 70-11
...mechanisms of endrin action, 63-16, 63-26
...organophosphate insecticides effects, 63-24, 69-19, 70-3
...Phosdrin effects on performance, 72-29, 73-3
...Phosdrin effects on vision, 73-4
...storage stability of human blood cholinesterase, 70-4
...toxic hazards, 62-8, 68-16, 78-31
...treatment of methamidophos poisoning, 78-26

Aerobatics

...blood donation effects, 84-4
...G effects on pilots, 72-28, 82-13

Aerospace

...medical screening guidance for commercial aerospace passengers, 06-1

Age

...age 60 rule, 94-20, 94-21, 94-22, 94-23, 04-8
...air traffic controller, health, 65-6, 71-8, 71-19, 72-20
 –performance, 61-1, 62-3, 65-21, 67-1, 71-36, 73-7, 84-6, 90-4
 –retirement age, 05-6, 05-22
...aircraft accident survival, 70-16
...aircraft accidents, pilots involved, 67-22, 70-18, 77-10, 95-11
...alcohol and altitude interaction, 88-2
...alcohol effects on performance, 95-3, 95-7
...aviation personnel, 64-1, 94-20, 94-21, 94-22, 94-23
...binocular fusion time effects, 66-35
...cardiovascular disease and performance, 64-4
...cardiovascular health changes in airmen, 72-26
...cockpit visual problems of senior pilots, 77-2, 77-7, 77-13, 77-14, 78-17
...complex monitoring performance effects, 81-12, 82-16, 83-15, 85-3, 88-2
...index for pilots, 77-6, 78-16, 78-27, 82-18
...pupillary reflex relationship, 65-25
...shiftwork, 95-19
...sonic boom effects during sleep, 72-19, 72-24, 72-35
...work capacity, 63-18, 63-33

Air ambulance

...cardiopulmonary factors in perinatal air transport, 82-5
...status of civilian air ambulance services, 71-18

Air bags

...restraint tests, 69-3, 69-4

Air loads

...effects on man, 63-9
...small-aircraft decompressions, 67-14

Air piracy

...deterrence, 78-35

Air traffic control

...ability requirements, 92-26, 98-8, 98-16
...Air Traffic Selection and Training (AT-SAT) project, 00-2, 06-16
...automation issues, 90-13, 92-31, 94-3, 95-4
...blink parameters and display highlighting, 99-8
...boredom with simulated radar control, 75-8, 80-1
...Cockpit Display of Traffic Information (CDTI), 00-30, 03-2, 03-13, 04-11
...cognitive style aspects, 99-12
...color highlighting and color deficiency, 92-6
...color use in ATC displays, 06-2, 06-6, 06-11, 06-15, 06-22
...communications, 96-10, 96-26, 98-17, 98-20, 99-21, 03-13, 05-19, 06-25
...conspicuity of colored and flashing targets, 90-3
 –target blink amplitudes, 97-10, 99-8
...density, warnings, and collision avoidance, 73-6

...flight progress strips, use of, 92-31, 94-3, 95-4, 95-9, 96-5, 00-5
...information complexity measures, implications for automation design, 04-17
...information requirements, TRACON, 95-16
...job task taxonomy, 93-1
...memory, 97-22
...napping and night shift performance, 00-10
...noise effects on performance of radar task, 79-24
...operational errors, evaluation of the Severity Index, 05-5
   −evaluation of HFACS and other models to describe causes, 05-25
   −review of human factors literature, 06-21
   −static sector characteristics, effect on, 06-4
...operational errors and incidences, causal factors and the JANUS technique, 03-21
   −development of temporal markers to profile, 06-20
   −role of shiftwork and fatigue, 99-2
...ophthalmic requirements, 96-12
...radar performance with and without a sweepline, 79-12.
   −with and without computer aiding, 89-1.
...radar training facility, 80-5, 80-15, 83-9
...resource management, crew, 95-21
...SATORI, 93-12, 97-13
...sector characteristics, activity and complexity, 06-29
   −static, and operational errors, 06-4
...selection and supervisory training, 92-16
...shiftwork, 71-2, 73-21, 73-22, 74-11, 75-7, 76-13, 77-23, 82-17
...situation assessment through re-creation of incidents (SATORI), 93-12, 98-14
...situation awareness, 94-27, 95-16, 97-13, 98-16, 99-3, 03-2, 03-5, 03-13, 04-11, 04-20
...simulator for research, 65-31
...systematic air traffic operations research initiative (SATORI), 97-13, 98-14
...teamwork, performance feedback in simulation, 00-25
   −teamwork, training platform, 99-24
...vigilance at three radar display target densities, 77-18
...vigilance of men and women on simulated radar task, 78-11, 80-17
...visual displays, cognitive complexity, 05-4
...visual taskload effects, on CFF change during complex monitoring, 85-13
   −on complex monitoring, 88-1, 90-3
...voice communications from, 93-20, 98-17, 98-20, 05-19

Air traffic controllers

...age and retirement, 05-6
...age effects on performance, 61-1, 62-3, 65-21, 67-1, 71-36, 73-7, 81-12, 82-16, 84-6, 90-4, 96-23, 99-18, 99-23, 05-6, 05-22
...aircraft mix and complexity ratings, 05-16
...anthropometry, 65-26
...anxiety with training, 89-7, 91-8
...anxiety with workload, 73-15, 80-14, 81-5
...aptitude tests for selection, 65-19, 68-14, 71-28, 71-36, 71-40, 72-18, 89-6, 90-8, 97-15, 98-23, 99-16, 00-2, 06-16
   −reweighting AT-SAT scores to reduce adverse impact, 06-16
...attitudes, 74-7, 74-12, 75-3, 79-11, 91-10, 00-17, 04-23
...attrition, 72-33, 74-2, 74-7, 75-3
...biochemical stress index, 74-11, 75-7, 77-23, 78-5, 78-40
...biodynamic evaluation, 71-8
...biographical factors associated with training success, 83-6, 84-6, 90-4, 94-13
...biomedical survey, 65-5, 65-6
...collegiate training initiative, 98-22
...color deficiency in a workforce sample, 06-1
...color perception and job performance, 83-11, 90-9, 92-6, 92-28, 92-29, 96-22, 06-2, 06-6, 06-11, 06-15, 06-22
...color vision tests, 85-7, 90-9, 92-28, 92-29, 95-13, 96-22, 04-10, 04-14, 06-2, 06-6, 06-11
...communication, 93-20, 95-15, 96-10, 96-20, 96-26, 98-17, 98-20, 99-21, 01-8, 01-9, 05-19, 06-25
...commuting (driving) risks before and after shifts, 06-13
...Composite Mood Adjective Check Lists to measure fatigue, 71-21
...disease incidence and prevalence, 78-21, 84-3
...education as selection factor, 76-6, 90-4
...experience as selection criterion, 63-31, 71-36, 74-8, 00-12
...fatigue and shiftwork, 99-2
   −and commuting risk factors before and after shifts, 06-13
...flight progress strips, use of, 92-31, 94-3, 95-4, 95-9, 96-5, 98-26, 00-5
...flight service station, training, 86-6, 91-4
   −organizational climate, 97-12
...headset interference tones, 92-4
...health changes, 71-19, 72-20, 78-39, 84-3
...height and weight data, errors in, 73-10
...incident reporting, 65-10, 03-19
...memory, 97-22, 98-16

...military experience and selection, 92-5
...motivational factors, 71-30, 73-2
...Multiple Task Performance Battery for selection, 72-5, 74-10
...Myers-Briggs personality types, 04-21
...napping and night shift performance, 00-10
...NEO Personality Inventory-Revised, compared with 16 PF test, 03-20
...occupational vision, 96-12, 96-27
...operational errors, evaluation of the Severity Index, 05-5
   –evaluation of HFACS and other models to describe causes, 05-25
   –static sector characteristics, influence on, 06-4
...operational errors/deviations, 99-2, 03-19, 03-21, 05-22, 06-21
...perceptions of aircraft performance, 00-24, 03-8, 05-16
...performance evaluation, 61-1, 65-22, 73-7, 93-12, 98-14, 00-2
...performance on radar monitoring tasks, 82-1, 83-13, 86-4, 88-1, 88-4. 90-3, 94-26, 95-23, 97-10, 98-16, 99-8
...performance during CDTI evaluation, 00-30, 03-2, 03-13
...personality factors, and disability retirement, 03-14
   –and performance, 70-14, 93-4, 94-13, 04-21
...physiological responses, 71-2, 73-21, 73-22, 74-11, 75-7, 76-13, 77-23, 82-17
...pilot satisfaction with services, 90-6
...presbyopic, 96-12, 96-27
...psychological testing, 61-1, 62-2, 80-14, 81-5, 92-30, 97-17, 98-23, 99-16, 99-23, 03-14, 03-20, 06-20
...selection, 62-2, 72-33, 74-8, 76-6, 77-25, 78-7, 78-36, 79-3, 79-14, 79-21, 80-7, 80-15, 80-17, 82-11, 83-6, 84-2, 84-6, 88-3, 89-6, 89-7, 90-4, 90-8, 90-13, 91-4. 91-8, 91-9, 91-18, 92-5, 92-26, 94-4, 94-8, 96-6, 96-13, 97-4, 97-15, 97-17, 97-19, 98-23, 99-16, 99-18, 99-23, 00-2, 00-12, 00-15, 03-20, 06-16
...sex differences in selection, training, and attrition, 72-22, 74-2, 74-7, 75-3, 96-13, 98-23
...shift rotation patterns, effects, 73-22, 75-7, 77-5, 85-2, 86-2, 95-12, 95-19, 96-23, 99-2, 00-10, 06-13
...situation awareness, 99-3, 03-2
...Sixteen Personality Factor test, air traffic controllers, 97-17, 03-20
...sleep patterns, 77-5, 95-12, 95-19, 00-10
...stress, 71-2, 73-21, 73-22, 74-11, 75-7, 76-13, 77-23, 80-14, 81-5, 82-17
...symptoms reported, 61-1

...taskload measures, 01-10, 02-2, 03-8, 05-16, 06-4, 06-29
...team work, performance feedback in simulation, 00-25
...training, 78-10, 79-3, 79-18, 80-5, 80-15, 82-2, 83-9, 88-3, 89-6, 89-7, 90-4, 90-8, 91-4, 94-9, 94-13, 95-4, 96-6, 98-8, 98-22, 98-23, 99-16, 00-12
...voice communications, 93-20, 95-15, 98-20, 99-21, 05-19

Air transportation

...animals, 77-8, 81-11, 84-5
...dry ice packaging in air cargo, sublimation rate, 06-19
...high risk pregnant women and neonates, 82-5, 00-33, 03-16
...human external loads, 98-13
...infectious disease substances, 95-29
...in-flight medical care, 00-13
...in-flight medical incapacitation and pilot impairment, 87-7, 04-16
...life preserver retrieval, , 03-9
...medical kits, 91-2, 91-3, 97-1, 00-13
...medical and psychological aspects, 71-10
...passenger safety information, availability, 04-19
...sports parachutists, restraint systems, 98-11
...standards for advanced systems, 71-33
...wheel-well stowaways, 96-25

Aircraft

...accident causes, 66-8, 66-25, 66-27, 66-29, 66-30, 67-23, 68-16, 69-2, 69-18, 71-9, 72-2, 73-5, 78-13, 78-31, 80-4, 82-15, 89-3, 98-5, 99-14, 99-15, 03-4, 04-4, 04-13, 04-24, 05-8, 06-7, 06-24
...accident investigation, 62-7, 62-9, 63-21, 63-35, 67-22, 69-18, 72-2, 73-5, 79-2, 79-6, 80-3, 80-6, 80-11, 81-10, 82-7, 83-8, 85-8, 97-21, 98-10, 99-11, 00-7, 00-22
...aging and maintenance, 92-3
...air flow and CFD prediction in a passenger cabin, 06-27
...attitude indicators, 73-9, 05-23
...aural glide slope cues for instrument approaches, 71-24
...biocidal fuel additive, 67-21
...cabin safety data bank, 79-23, 82-8
...cabin safety subject index, 84-1, 85-1
...cabin ventilation flow fields, 04-7, 06-27
   –decontamination with vaporized hydrogen peroxide, 06-10
...cargo compartment environment, 81-11
...checklists, 91-7
...cockpit delethalization, 66-3, 66-12, 71-3, 72-6, 72-7, 72-15

...cockpit visual problems, 77-2, 77-7, 77-13, 77-14, 78-17, 03-12
...communication in light aircraft, 72-31
...computational fluid dynamics (CFD) in predicting pathogen distribution in a passenger cabin, 06-27
...contaminant distribution prediction in a passenger cabin, 06-27
...control forces and female pilots, 72-27, 73-23
...crew smoke-protective devices, 76-5, 78-4, 83-14, 89-5, 89-8, 89-11
...decompression hazards, 67-14, 70-12, 99-4
...decontamination of passenger cabin, 06-10
...design changes to reduce injuries, 71-3, 72-7, 83-8
...displays, 98-9, 98-12, 03-2, 03-5, 03-13, 04-5, 05-23
...ditching studies, 78-1, 91-6, 98-19, 04-12
...escape slides, studies of, 98-3, 99-10
...evacuation, 62-9, 65-7, 66-42, 70-16, 70-19, 72-30, 77-11, 78-3, 78-23, 79-5, 79-6, 80-12, 81-7, 89-5, 89-12, 92-27, 95-22, 95-25, 96-18, 98-19, 99-10, 99-30, 00-11, 01-18, 03-15, 04-2, 04-12, 05-2
...exits, size of in evacuation, 99-10, 04-12
...evacuation models, 94-11, 97-20
...fire, smoke protection after accidents, 67-4, 70-16, 70-20, 78-4, 83-10, 85-10, 89-5, 89-8, 89-11, 89-12
...fire vs. no fire on rotorcraft accidents, 05-17
...fires, toxicity of combustion products, 71-41, 77-9, 85-5, 86-1, 86-3, 86-5, 89-4, 91-17, 95-8
...flight inspection, evaluation, 95-18
...flight manuals, 91-7
...flight training devices, 94-25, 95-6
...floor proximity marking systems, 98-2
...GPS displays, 98-9, 98-12, 99-9, 99-13, 99-26, 00-4, 03-17
...head impact kinematics, 92-20
...Highway-in-the Sky (HITS) display, 00-31
...inspection, 89-9, 94-12, 95-14
  –visual standards used for inspectors, 05-21
...instrument display, 75-12, 98-28, 00-8, 00-31
...interior wall padding and neck injury potential, 93-14
...landing, simulated night approaches, 77-12, 78-15, 79-4, 81-6
...life preserver retrieval, 03-9
...maintenance, 89-9, 90-14, 91-16, 92-3, 93-5, 93-15, 94-12, 95-14, 95-31, 96-2, 05-21
...medical incidents inflight, 00-13
...neck injury potential, 93-14
...NEXRAD display, 04-5
...noise effects measurement, 71-1, 72-32
...noise effects on birds, 62-4
...noise levels, 68-21, 68-25, 70-6

  –and pilot hearing thresholds, 05-21
...nongyropscopic blind flight instrument, 66-32
...oxygen system design, 78-9, 04-3
...ozone concentrations and effects, 79-20, 80-9, 89-13
...padding for crash protection, 66-40
...performance characteristics, perceived by ATCSs, 00-24, 03-8
...propeller paint schemes conspicuity, 78-29
...radioactive material shipments, 82-12
...readability of emergency signs in smoke, 79-22
...restraint installation, 66-33, 67-13, 72-15
...restraint system evaluation, 69-3, 69-4, 69-5, 71-12, 72-3, 72-6, 78-6, 78-12, 78-24, 79-17, 80-3, 81-10, 82-7, 94-19, 95-2, 95-30, 98-11, 99-5
...seat cushion flotation, 66-13, 98-19
...seat evaluation, 78-6, 78-24, 79-17, 80-3, 81-10, 82-7, 83-3, 90-11
...seat impact injuries, 66-18, 72-15, 89-3
...simulator operation using drugs, 64-18
...SST anticollision lights, 70-9, 70-15, 71-42
...stall warning device, 66-31
...standards for advanced aerospace systems, 71-33
...sunscreen-treated windows, 78-28
...toxicity of engine oil thermal degradation, 83-12
...unmanned aircraft, 04-24, 06-8
...warning signals and pilot hearing thresholds, 05-12
...water spray system, 98-4
...wheel-well passengers, 96-25

Airport

...cues for approach and landing, 79-4, 79-25, 81-6, 82-6
...medical services, 65-3, 71-10
...precautionary emergency evacuation data, 99-30

Airway facilities personnel

...human factors, 94-5
...job attitudes, 77-21, 79-11, 83-7

Airway Science Curriculum Demonstration Project

...air traffic control specialists, 91-18
...initial evaluation, 88-5

Airworthiness Inspectors

...assessment of job performance, 87-4

Alcohol

...alcoholic airline pilot rehabilitation, 85-12
...altitude effects, on blood levels, 70-5
  –on performance, 68-18, 79-26, 82-3, 85-5, 88-2
...ataxia test battery effects, 79-9
...complex performance effects, 66-29, 69-14, 72-4, 79-7, 85-5, 88-2, 94-24, 95-3, 95-7

...congener effects, 79-7, 79-9
...detection methods, 83-2, 91-12, 04-13
...disorientation-related responses, 71-6, 71-16, 71-20, 71-34, 71-39, 72-34
...findings in general aviation accidents, 66-27, 66-29, 68-16, 69-2, 78-31, 80-4, 95-28, 98-5, 04-13, 05-20
...hangover effects, 79-7, 79-26
...instrument flight performance effects, 72-4
...low doses and performance, 94-24, 95-3, 95-7
...postmortem in fatal accidents, 92-24, 98-5, 00-21, 03-18, 04-4, 04-13, 05-20
...problem solving effects, 72-11
...readiness to perform testing, 93-13, 95-24
...tests for alcoholism after intoxication in non-alcoholics, 83-2
...thalamic activity effects, 78-2
...visual functions effects, 78-2, 79-15

Altitude

...alcohol effects, 68-18, 79-26, 82-3, 85-5, 88-2
...antihistamine effects on performance, 68-15
...antihistamine-decongestant preparations effects, 78-19, 78-20
...blood alcohol levels effects, 70-5
...blood donation effects on tolerance, 84-4
...chamber reactions, 77-4, 90-12
...civilian training need, 91-13, 03-10
...cosmic radiation, at SST altitudes, 71-26, 80-2
...cosmic radiation, crewmembers and passengers, 92-2, 00-33, 03-16, 05-14
  –SST altitudes, 71-26, 80-2
...decompression hazards, 67-14, 70-12, 99-4
...decompression, performance after, 66-10
...heat effects on performance, 71-17
...human tolerance, 62-6
...marihuana effects on performance, 75-6
...oxygen masks, efficiency of, 62-21, 66-7, 66-9, 66-20, 67-3, 67-9, 72-10, 79-13, 80-18, 85-10, 89-10, 93-6, 98-27
...oxygen need, 66-28, 78-9
...ozone concentrations and effects, 79-20, 80-9
...penetrating eye injuries effects, 62-12
...performance effects, 66-15, 71-11, 82-3, 82-4, 82-10, 83-15, 85-3, 85-5, 88-2, 97-7, 97-9
...portable oxygen system, 98-27.
...propranolol effects on tolerance, 79-10, 80-10
...smokers, effects on, 97-7
...tolerance after crash diet, 81-2, 81-8
...tolerance of beta blocked hypertensives, 92-19
...tolerance with pulmonary disease, 77-16
...tolerance with sickle cell trait, 76-15, 78-30
...visual fields effects on glaucoma patients and the elderly, 91-1
...work tolerance effects, 63-33, 82-3
...wheel-well stowaways, 96-25

Animal transportation

...freezing and subfreezing temperature effects on dogs, 87-3
...heat and humidity effects on dogs, 77-8, 81-11, 84-5, 87-8

Anthropometry

...forensic, 79-2
...adult face, 78-14, 93-10
...adult female, 83-16
...air traffic controllers, 65-26
...center of gravity, 62-14, 65-23, 69-22
...faces of children for oxygen mask design, 66-9
...female crewmember facial anthropometry, 83-14
...flight attendants, 75-2, 75-13
...flight inspection pilots and technicians, 95-18
...head and face of adults, 93-10
...human pelvis, 82-9
...shoulder slope, 65-14
...weight distribution when sitting, 62-1

Anthropomorphic dummies

...criteria for crashworthiness, 96-11
...design, 82-9, 83-16
...evaluation, 78-6, 78-24, 79-17, 83-3
...3- and 6-year-old dummies, 76-9
...thoracic mass, determination, 96-7

Anticollision lights

...effects of backscatter, 72-8
...exposure effects under simulated IFR conditions, 66-39
...SST, 70-9, 70-15, 71-42

Aphakia

...accident risk assessment, 95-11
...incidence in airmen, 91-14, 92-14

Arousal

...by distracting stimuli, 71-7
...nystagmus effects, 62-17
...simulated radar control task, 75-8, 77-18, 81-12, 88-1
...vestibular responses effects, 63-29

Attention

...anticollision observing responses, 73-6
...auditory distraction effects, 72-14
...conspicuity of flashing and color targets, 90-3
  –target blink amplitude, 97-10, 99-8
...personality and physiological correlates, 73-14
...self-estimates of distractibility, 72-25
...psychophysiological indices, 99-28

...simulated radar task, 77-18, 78-11, 79-12, 80-17, 81-12, 82-1, 82-16, 86-4, 88-1, 89-1
...switching in readiness to perform, 95-24
...time-sharing ability, 76-1, 78-33
...visual taskload effects on CFF change during complex monitoring, 85-13
...visual taskload effects on complex monitoring, 88-1, 90-3, 94-26, 95-23, 96-9, 99-28

Audiology

...advanced and ATC selection, 90-13
...auditory fatigue, 63-19, 65-1, 65-2
...binaural beat perception, 63-17
...cockpit noise intensities, 68-21, 68-25
...ear-protector ratings, 73-20, 75-11
...earphone transient response, 63-7
...hearing threshold, pilots vs. non-pilots, 05-12
...interaural intensity difference limen, 67-10
...noise audiometry, 71-1
...noise effects on aircrew personnel, 72-32
...speech intelligibility improvement, 70-6, 72-31, 73-13, 76-3
...table of intensity increments, 66-4
...temporary threshold shift, 79-16

Automation

...advanced, and ATCS selection, 90-13, 92-26, 97-19, 98-23
...boredom and monotony as stressors, 80-1
...complacency on radar monitoring task, 82-1
...complex monitoring performance predictors, 80-17, 86-4
...flight progress strips, 92-31, 94-3, 95-8, 96-5
...general aviation, pilot responses to autopilot malfunctions, 97-24
...information complexity measures and design implications, 04-17
...physiological stress in controllers, 82-17
...radar performance with and without computer aiding, 89-1
...recovery of radar monitoring performance following startle, 83-13
...visual taskload effects on CFF change during complex monitoring, 85-13
...visual taskload effects on complex monitoring, 88-1

Aviation maintenance

...human factors, 89-9, 90-14, 91-16, 92-3, 93-5, 93-15, 94-12, 95-31, 96-2
...visual standards and tests used for inspectors, 05-21

Aviation medical examiners

...and drug testing program, 92-15

...exams of first-class certificate holders by senior AMEs, 71-38
...performance, 84-7

Ballistocardiography

...bibliography, 65-15
...research and current status, 64-12
...stroke volume relationship, 65-8

Behavioral types

...coronary-prone Type A and complex monitoring performance, 86-4
...Type A and ATCS training performance, 94-13

Benzodiazepines

...analysis in forensic urine samples, 96-14

Birds

...possible sonotropic effects of a commercial air transport, 62-4

Blood

...altitude effects on alcohol levels, 70-5
...autoregulation of renal flow, 63-32
...cerebrovascular disease detection, 65-4
...cholinesterase measurement, 67-5
...clot dissolution therapy, 64-5
...comparison of serum cholinesterase methods, 70-13, 72-12
...cyanide, 94-7
...donation effects, 84-4
...erythrocyte volume spectra, 63-8
...gene expression profiles, maintenance after blood storage, 04-1
...hemoconcentration with endrin poisoning, 66-11
...oxygen saturation, 66-7, 66-15, 66-20, 67-3, 67-9
...phospholipids, 71-2, 73-21, 73-22
...plasma catecholamine determination, 66-6, 71-15
...pressure changes, in ATC population, 71-19, 72-20, 78-39, 84-3
 –in third-class certificate holders, 72-26
...pressure levels of active pilots, 84-3
...pressures by rapid indirect method, 70-21
...pulmonary flow with glyceryl trinitrate, 64-11
...pulmonary thromboembolism, 64-7
...sickle cell disease and trait, 76-15, 78-30, 80-20
...storage stability of human blood cholinesterases, 70-4
...tests for alcohol abuse, 83-2

Cabin safety

...cabin simulator, experimental, 97-18
...cabin ventilation flow fields, 04-7, 06-27
 –decontamination with vaporized hydrogen peroxide, 06-10

...computer evacuation models, 94-11, 97-20
...data bank, 79-23, 82-8
...passenger safety information, availability, 04-19
...subject index, 84-1, 85-1

Caloric irrigation

...after habituation to rotation, 63-13
...alcohol effect on response, 71-6
...arousal effects on nystagmus, 62-17
...elicitation of secondary nystagmus, 63-3
...nystagmus after habituation, 63-14, 64-14, 65-19, 67-2

Canes

...used by blind passengers, 80-12

Carbon monoxide

...carboxyhemoglobin standards, 98-21
...cause of aircraft accidents, 68-16, 69-2, 82-15, 00-9, 05-9
...levels in aircraft accident victims, 70-16, 80-11, 00-9
...relative toxic hazards of materials, 77-9
...times to incapacitation of rats, 89-4, 93-7

Cardiovascular

...age and physical training effects, 63-18, 64-1
...antihistamine-decongestant preparations effects, 78-20
...ballistocardiographic research, 64-12, 65-8, 65-15
...blood donation effects, 84-4
...blood pressure measurement, 66-16, 66-36, 70-21, 84-3
...cerebrovascular disease detection, 65-4
...changes in ATC population, 71-19, 72-20, 78-39, 84-3
...changes in third-class certificate holders, 72-26
...coronary heart disease detection, 74-6, 78-38
...dextroamphetamine effects on heart rates, 75-14
...endrin effects, 63-16, 66-11
...evaluation with treadmill and step test, 64-3
...function in aviation stress protocol, 78-5
...glyceryl trinitrate effects on pulmonary vasculature, 64-11
...health, age, and performance, 64-4
...heart rates during instrument approaches, 70-7, 71-24, 75-12
...heart rates in air tanker pilots, 68-26
...heart rates in ATCSs, 71-2, 73-21, 73-22, 74-11
...heart rates in student pilots, 67-15, 69-12
...heart rates with complex vigilance tasks, 69-8, 75-8, 86-4
...heart rates with simulated sonic booms, 71-29
...in-flight incapacitation, 87-7

...physiological responses on cross-country flights, 71-23
...post mortem findings after accidents, 69-18, 80-8, 85-6
...prediction of heart rates under stress, 69-7
...prevalence among civil airmen, 89-2
...problems associated with aviation safety, 78-38
...recognition of posterior infarction, 64-19
...rehabilitation after infarction, 64-2, 66-17, 66-21
...responses to hyperpyrexia, 64-8
...rheoencephalography and cerebrovascular disease, 65-4, 67-11
...risk factors, 90-7
...startle effects on heart rates, 69-21
...stress effects on heart rates, 68-17
...thromboembolic disease treatment, 64-5
...transducer for heart sounds, 68-3

Case reports

...ethanol origin in postmortem urine, 04-13
...in-flight loss of consciousness, 63-21
...insecticide exposure, 63-24
...methamphetamine involvement in a pilot fatality, 03-22
...physical conditioning after infarction, 66-21
...pulmonary thromboembolism, 64-7
...quinine elimination, 94-16
...rheoencephalography in cerebrovascular disease detection, 65-4
...seizures inflight, 64-6

Center of gravity

...adults, 62-14
...children, 65-23
...infants, 69-22

Certification, aeromedical

...airmen attrition, 72-13, 73-8
...alcoholic airline pilots rehabilitation, 85-12
...analysis of denial actions, 68-9, 74-5, 76-10, 78-25, 80-19, 83-5, 84-9, 85-9, 86-7, 90-5
...aphakia, 91-14, 92-14, 93-11, 95-11
...aviation medical examiner performance, 84-7
...color vision, tests, 67-8, 83-11, 85-7, 90-9, 93-17, 95-13, 96-22
 –X-Chrom lens, 78-22
...contact lens use, 90-10, 00-18
...diabetic conditions, glucose concentrations in transportation accidents, 00-22
...disease prevalence and incidence, 73-8, 81-9, 84-8, 89-2, 90-7
...errors in height and weight data, 73-10
...estimate of active airmen, 68-5
...exams of first-class certificate holders by senior AMEs, 71-38

...gender differences in refractive surgery, 00-23
...glare, 94-15
...glaucoma, 91-1
...intraocular implants, 92-14, 93-11
...medications found in postmortem and medical history, 06-12
...neuropsychological screening of airmen, 92-11
...photorefractive keratectomy, 98-25
...procedures, 71-25, 82-14
...refractive surgery, 00-19, 00-23, 06-9
 –gender differences, 00-23
 –radial keratectomy, 98-25, 00-19, 06-9
 –radial keratotomy, 99-6, 00-19, 06-9
...rheoencephalography and cerebrovascular disease, 65-4, 67-11
...sickle cell disease and trait, 76-15, 80-20
...suicides, aircraft-assisted in general aviation pilots, drug involvement, 06-5
...tests for alcohol abuse, 83-2
...vision restrictions and pilot demographics, 04-6
...vision standards and screening tests used with aircraft maintenance personnel, 05-21

Charts

...readability, 77-13, 78-17

Circadian periodicity

...bibliography of shiftwork research, 83-17
...disruption of intercontinental flights, 65-16, 65-28, 65-29, 65-30, 68-8, 69-17
...effects of shifts in wake-sleep cycle, 75-10, 76-11, 86-2
...excretion of magnesium and calcium, 68-4
...rotating shiftwork, 86-2, 99-2

Civil Aeromedical Institute (CAMI)

...historical vignettes, prefaces to 87-1, 97-1, 98-1, 01-1, 03-1
...history of aeromedical research contributions, 05-3

Clothing

...effects on drag forces, 63-9

Cold

...effect on dogs shipped by air transport, 87-3
...effect on manual performance, 68-13
...exposure after water spray, 98-4
...skin temperature to predict tolerance, 71-4
...thermal balance, 66-23
...thermal protection by life preservers, 85-11

Color

...air traffic control displays, status of, 06-11
...conspicuity of radar targets, 90-3
...highlighting targets, 92-6

Color vision

...air traffic control specialists performance, 83-11, 06-6, 06-11, 06-15, 06-22
...air traffic control workgroup sample, 06-2
...clinical tests as predictors of practical tests, 73-18, 75-1, 92-28, 92-29, 95-13, 96-22, 04-9
...defective, and color highlighting, 92-6
 –and radar displays, 06-22
 –and signal lights, recognition, 71-27, 71-32
...impairment by sunscreen materials, 78-28
...tests, 67-8, 85-7, 90-9, 93-17, 95-13, 96-22
 –tests used for maintenance inspectors, 05-21
...test illuminant, 93-16
...X-Chrom lens for improving, 78-22

Communication

...ATC/pilot, CDTI effects, 03-13, 04-11
 –voice, 93-20, 95-15, 96-26, 98-17, 98-20, 99-21, 05-19, 06-25
...binaural beat perception, 63-17
...earphone response, 63-7
...interaural intensity difference limen, 67-10
...light aircraft, 72-31
...organizational, and technology change, 99-25
...predictor for empowerment, 98-24
...role in aircraft maintenance and inspection, 90-10
...role in promoting change within Airway Facilities Service, 83-7
...speech intelligibility improvement, 70-6, 72-31, 73-13, 76-3
...table of intensity increments, 66-4
...tactile, 62-11, 62-16
...voice, methods and metrics, 96-10, 96-20, 06-25

Contact lenses

...epidemiological study of certification, 90-10
...monovision and airline accident, 00-18

Cosmic radiation

...air carrier crew, exposure of, 80-2, 92-2, 00-33, 03-16, 05-14

Crashworthiness

...dummy criteria, 96-11
...energy-absorbing seat effectiveness, 83-3, 90-11
...head impact and interior walls, 92-20, 93-14
...occupant survival in general aviation accidents, 81-10, 82-7, 83-8, 98-3

Deceleration

...bibliography, 63-30
...cockpit delethalization, 66-3, 66-12, 72-6, 72-7, 72-15, 81-10
...head impacts while wearing restraint systems, 72-6

...human tolerance, 62-6, 83-3
...illumination effects during angular deceleration, 68-28
...impact injuries in pregnancy, 68-6, 68-24
...kinematics of human body, 62-13
...padding for crash protection, 66-40
...rearward-facing seats, 69-13
...restraint systems, 67-13, 69-3, 69-4, 69-5, 69-13, 72-3, 72-15, 80-3, 81-10, 82-7, 83-8, 99-5
...seat impact injuries, 66-18, 72-15, 81-10, 82-7
...side-facing seats, 69-13
...survival of extreme vertical impacts, 62-19
...survival of free-fall impacts, 63-15
...survival of water impacts, 65-12
...tolerances of face, 65-20

Decision-making

...employee participation in, 91-10, 92-13, 92-17
..."expert" pilot model, 97-6
...perceptions of aircraft performance characteristics by ATCSs, 00-24
...personal minimums tool, 96-19, 98-6
...skills in pilots, 98-7
...training in pilots, 87-6, 96-19, 98-6
...weather information, use of, 97-3, 97-23, 04-5
...willingness to take off into marginal weather, 05-7, 05-15

Decompression

...altitude chamber experience, 77-4, 90-12
...effects on performance, 66-10
...effects of propranolol on TUF, 79-10, 80-10
...need for civilian training, 91-13, 03-10
...oxygen mask evaluation, 66-20, 67-3, 72-10, 79-13, 80-18, 96-4, 98-27, 00-6
...pressurized small aircraft, 67-14
...supersonic transports, 99-4
...tolerable profiles for SST, 70-12

Depth perception

...general, 62-15, 63-10, 63-20, 63-28, 64-13, 65-11, 65-32, 66-22, 66-24, 67-18, 67-20
...light adaptation device, 66-38
...monovision contact lenses in airline accident, 00-18

Diet

...human tolerance, effects, 81-2
...performance, effects, 81-8

Disorientation

...accidents due to, 78-13, 95-1, 96-21
...adaptation, 65-18, 65-24, 66-37, 67-2, 67-6, 67-7, 67-12, 67-19, 68-2, 68-28, 69-20, 74-3
...alcohol effects, 71-6, 71-16, 71-20, 71-34, 71-39, 72-34
...familiarization techniques, 70-17, 77-24
...visually induced, 69-23, 70-2, 71-22

Distraction

...auditory distraction and performance, 72-14
...susceptibility, measurement of, 72-25

Ditching

...flotation and survival equipment studies, 78-1, 85-11, 03-9, 04-12
...frequency of occurrence, 98-19
...infant flotation device, 71-37, 91-6
...seat cushion flotation, 66-13, 95-20
...water survival training programs, 98-19

DNA

...detection of postmortem alcohol-producing microorganisms, 00-16
...identification of forensic specimens, 06-14
...profiling for quality assurance, 98-18, 99-14

Drugs

...aircraft accidents, role of, 68-16, 78-31, 85-8, 92-23, 94-14, 95-28, 96-14, 97-14, 98-10, 98-18, 99-29, 00-20, 00-21, 03-7, 05-20
 –quality assurance of forensic findings, 99-11, 99-15, 04-15
...antihistamine effects, at altitude, 68-15, 78-19, 78-20
 –on cognitive performance, 99-20
 –on shiftwork performance, 97-25
...antimotion sickness, 81-16, 82-19
...atropine, and performance, 93-19
 –and Phosdrin effects on vision, 73-4
...benzodiazepines, forensic analysis, 96-14
...butalbital, forensic analysis, 00-29
...cocaine, forensic analysis, 03-23, 03-24
...chlordimeform toxicity, 77-19
...chlorpheniramine, forensic analysis, 99-29
...complex performance effects, 69-9
...detection and identification, 92-25, 96-17, 97-14, 98-18, 04-15, 05-8, 05-10, 05-11, 05-20, 06-3, 06-12, 06-17
...dextroamphetamine, effects during angular acceleration, 73-17, 76-12
 –effects during sleep loss, 75-14
...enantiomeric analysis of ephedrines and norephedrines, 05-8
...fatigue, and use, 63-12, 75-14
...glyceryl trinitrate effects on pulmonary vasculature, 64-11
...lithium carbonate effects on performance, 77-17
...marihuana, 73-12, 85-8

...marihuana and altitude effects on performance, 75-6
...melatonin, 98-10
...methamidophos poisoning, 78-26
...methamphetamine, forensic finding, 03-22
...opiate determination (vs. poppy seed use) in post-mortem sample, 05-11
...orthostatic tolerance effects, 63-34
...performance effects in aircraft simulator, 64-18
...post-mortem findings and medical history, 06-12
...propranolol, effects on altitude tolerance, 79-10, 80-10
 –quantitation, 05-10
...readiness to perform testing, 93-13
...secobarbital effects during angular acceleration, 73-17
...selegiline metabolites, 97-14
...sildenafil (Viagra), method for detecting in postmortem samples, 00-20, 06-3
...testing programs and AMEs, 92-15
...tranquilizer, effects on body temperature, 63-23, 66-14
 –use in flight training, 69-12
...triamterene in fatal accident, 92-13
...Vardenafil (Levitra), method for detecting in post-mortem samples, 06-17
...visual reflexes effects, 79-15
...work capacity effects, 63-34

Earphones

...headset interference tones, 92-4
...transient response, 63-7

Earplugs

...ratings, 73-20, 75-11

Education

...aviation medical examiners, 84-7
...factor, in air traffic controller selection, 76-6, 96-6
 –in air traffic controller success, 76-6, 83-6

Electrocardiogram

...amplitude/frequency analysis, 74-6
...diagnosis of posterior infarction, 64-19

Energy

...cost of treadmill work, 62-5
...energy-absorbing seat effectiveness, 83-3, 90-11

Environment

...aerospace, commercial passengers, medical screening guidance, 06-1
...cabin ventilation, flow fields, 04-7
 –computational fluid dynamics for predictions, 06-27
 –decontamination with vaporized hydrogen peroxide, 06-10
...cargo compartments, 81-11
...effects of mass air transportation, 71-10

Equipment

...air traffic control displays and color vision, 06-2, 06-6, 06-11, 06-15, 06-22
...air traffic situation assessment (SATORI), 93-12
...alcohol detection, 91-12
...anthropometry in design, 65-26, 75-2
...anticollision lights, 66-39, 70-9, 70-15, 71-42, 72-8
...ARTS-III effects on controller stress, 76-13
...attitude indicators, equivalence tests, 05-23
...automation design, measures of information complexity, 04-17
...blood pressure measurement, 66-16, 70-21
...Cockpit Display of Traffic Information (CDTI), 00-30, 03-2, 03-5, 03-13, 04-11, 04-20
...compact instrument display, 75-12
...crew smoke-protective devices, 76-5, 78-4, 78-41, 83-14, 89-8, 89-11, 05-18
...disorientation familiarization, 70-17
...Emergency Escape Breathing Device, 92-18
...emergency lighting, 66-42, 79-22, 80-13, 81-7
...escape slides, strength, 98-3
...evaporative water loss, 67-17
...fire, smoke protection, 67-4, 70-20, 78-4, 83-10, 85-10, 89-5, 89-8, 89-11, 89-12, 05-18
...flotation and survival, 78-1, 85-11
...GPS displays, 98-8, 98-12, 99-9, 99-13, 99-26, 00-4, 03-17
...head injury criteria (HIC) test component test device, evaluation, 04-18
...head-up displays, 98-28
...Highway-in-the-Sky (HITS) display, 00-31
...infant flotation device, 71-37, 91-6
...instrument readability by senior pilots, 77-2, 77-7
...lapbelt restraint in pregnancy, 68-24
...life preserver retrieval, 03-9
...light adaptation device, 66-38
...medical kits, 91-2, 91-3, 00-13, 00-13
...NEXRAD display, 04-5
...nongyroscopic blind flight instrument, 66-32
...oxygen, 62-21, 66-7, 66-9, 66-10, 66-20, 67-3, 67-9, 72-10, 78-4, 79-13, 80-18, 83-10, 85-10, 89-5, 89-10, 93-6, 95-17, 96-4, 98-27, 00-6, 04-3
...padding for crash protection, 66-40
...performance testing, 66-19
...personnel lifting devices, rotorcraft, 98-13
...protective, for aircraft accidents, 65-7, 66-3, 66-12
...restraint systems, 67-13, 69-3, 69-4, 69-5, 72-3, 72-6, 83-8, 94-19, 99-5

...seat cushion flotation, 66-13
...secondary container alternative for transportation of infectious substances, 95-29
...stall warning, 66-31
...transducer, 68-3
...upper torso restraint acceptance, 71-12
...visual displays, methods to assess complexity in air traffic control, 05-4

Evacuation, passenger emergency

...acoustic signals for exit location, 79-5
...air carrier accidents, 62-9, 65-7, 70-16
...bibliography, 63-30
...blind passengers, 80-12
...cabin simulator, experimental, 97-18
...children, 66-42, 01-18
...computer models, 94-11
...ditching (evacuation into water), simulated, 04-12
...Emergency Escape Breathing Device, 92-18
...emergency lighting, aisle seat arm rests, 81-7
 –exit signs, 79-22, 80-13, 81-7
 –floor, 98-2
...escape slides and platforms, 96-18, 98-3
...handicapped passengers, 77-11
...history of smoke/fume protective breathing equipment, 87-5
...human external loads, 98-13
...infants, 66-42, 01-18, 05-2
...injuries, 79-6, 79-23, 82-8, 99-30, 03-15
...motivation of passengers, 96-18, 04-2
...passenger flow rates between compartments, 78-3
...passenger safety information, availability, 04-19
...passenger workload and protective breathing, 87-2, 89-5
...precautionary, 99-30, 00-11
...railroad accident, 73-1
...readability of emergency signs in smoke, 79-22, 80-13, 81-7
...seating configuration, 89-14, 92-27, 95-22, 03-15
...simulation by computer models, 72-30, 78-23, 94-11, 97-20
 –experimental cabin, 97-18
...SST mockup tests, 70-19
...size of exits in evacuation, 99-10, 04-12
...tests using L-1649, 66-42
...tests using protective smoke hood, 70-20, 89-12, 05-18
...type III exits, 92-27, 95-22, 95-25, 03-15, 04-2
...water survival training programs analysis, 98-19

Exercise

...auscultatory and intra-aortic pressures, 66-36
...human tolerances, effects on, 82-4, 82-10
...magnesium and calcium excretion, effects on, 68-4

...myocardial infarction, before and after, 64-2
 –effects after, 66-17, 66-21
...tolerance at altitude, 63-33
...treadmill work, energy cost of, 62-5
...air traffic controller selection, 63-31, 74-8, 78-7, 83-6
...ATCS, correlation with age and performance, 67-1, 73-7
...pilots in general aviation accidents, 77-10
...relation to reported symptoms of ATCSs, 65-6

Eye

...age and binocular fusion time, 66-35
...airman visual acuity, midair collisions, 75-5
...alcohol effects on eye movements, 72-34
...anticollision lights, 66-39, 70-9, 70-15, 71-42, 72-8
...aphakia, prevalence in civil airmen, 91-14, 92-14, 93-11
...bifocal effects on radar monitoring, 82-16
...bright lights and visual disturbances during nighttime flight operations, 06-28
...contact lenses, 90-10, 00-18
...cockpit visual problems of senior pilots, 77-2, 77-7, 77-13, 77-14, 78-17
...color vision and signal lights, 71-27, 71-32, 73-18, 75-1, 78-22, 93-17, 04-14, 06-2
...color vision tests, for ATCS, 83-11, 85-7, 90-9, 92-28, 92-29, 95-13, 96-22, 04-10, 04-14
 –for aviation maintenance inspectors, 05-21
...depth perception, 63-10, 63-28, 67-20, 00-18
...equidistance tendency, 65-11
...fatigue effects on binocular fusion time, 69-1
...glare tests, 94-15
...glaucoma, visual field and altitude, 91-1
...laser light illumination, effects on simulator performance, 03-12, 04-9
 –incidence during flights, 06-23
...lateral movements in student pilots, 67-15
...movements during simulated air traffic control, 94-26, 95-23, 96-9
...neural control of ciliary muscle, 63-5
...occupational vision, en route centers, 96-12, 96-27
...optokinetic stimulation, 70-2, 70-10, 71-22
...pathology in accident airmen, 81-14, 83-18
...penetrating injuries, 62-12
...photic stimulation, 66-39
...photorefractive keratectomy, 98-25
...pilot demographics and vision restrictions, 04-6
...propeller paint schemes conspicuity, 78-29
...pupillary movement with fatigue, 65-9
...pupillary reflex with age, 65-25
...radial keratectomy, 98-25, 00-19, 06-9
...radial keratotomy, 99-6, 00-19, 06-9

...reaction time, flash luminance and duration, 67-24
...refractive surgery and aeromedical certification, 00-19, 06-9
...senior pilots, cockpit visual problems, 77-2, 77-7, 77-13, 77-14, 78-17
...simulation of objects moving in depth, 65-32
...size and distance perception, 62-15, 64-13, 66-22, 66-24, 67-18
...spatial extent, perception of, 63-20
...spiral aftereffect test, 64-9, 64-10, 64-17, 68-10, 69-15, 71-31
...target detection, highlighted, 97-10, 99-8
...tests for color vision, 67-8, 83-11, 93-16, 93-17, 06-2
  –tests for aviation maintenance inspectors, 05-21
...two-flash thresholds, 68-20, 70-15, 71-42
...vision through sunscreen materials, 78-28
...visually induced disorientation, 69-23, 70-2, 71-22
...X-Chrom lens for improving color vision, 78-22

Fatigue

...air tanker pilots, 68-26
...antihistamine-decongestant preparations effects, 78-20
...auditory, 63-19, 65-1, 65-2
...aviation activities, 65-13, 81-13
...binocular fusion time effects, 69-1
...Composite Mood Adjective Check Lists to measure in ATCSs, 71-21
...8- vs. 10-hr. work schedules, 95-32
...eye blink-rate measures, 94-17, 94-26, 99-28
...intercontinental jet flights, 65-16, 65-28, 65-29, 65-30, 68-8, 69-17
...mitigation with Spartase, 63-12
...plasma catecholamine determination, 66-6, 71-15
...pupillary movement with, 65-9
...readiness to perform testing, 93-13, 95-24
...shiftwork, rotating, 86-2, 99-2
  –effects on commuting risk factors before and after shift, 06-13
  –effects on wake-sleep cycle, 75-10, 76-11, 85-2, 95-12, 95-19
...sleep deprivation effects, 70-8, 75-14, 85-3
...tolerance after crash diet, 81-2
...tolerance after exercise, 82-4, 82-10
...visual, during vigilance task, 94-26, 96-9
...visual taskload effects on CFF change during complex monitoring, 85-13

Federal Air Surgeon

...review of 1966 program, 67-25
...review of 1976 program, 76-8

Fire

...crew smoke-protective devices, 76-5, 78-4, 78-14, 78-41, 83-14, 05-18
...effects in air carrier accidents, 62-9, 65-7, 70-16
...flammability of toiletries in oxygen, 63-27
...passenger protective breathing devices, 67-4, 70-20, 83-10, 85-10, 87-2, 87-5, 89-5, 89-8, 89-11, 89-12, 05-18
...smoke effects on identifying emergency signs, 79-22, 80-13, 81-7
...toxicity of products in aircraft fires, 7 1-41, 77-9, 85-5, 86-1, 86-3, 86-5, 89-4, 90-15, 90-16
...toxicity of seat fire-blocking materials, 86-1
...vs. non-fire, forensics, 00-9, 05-9
  –in rotorcraft accidents, 05-17

Flight attendants

...anthropometry, 75-2
...functional strength, 75-13
...injuries, cabin safety data bank, 79-23, 82-8
...ozone effects, 79-20
...water survival training programs, 98-19

Flotation devices

...infant, 91-6
...life preserver retrieval, 03-9

...methods of seat cushion use, 95-20
...personal devices, 98-19

Forensics (See Toxicology)

Fuel

...biocidal additive, 67-21

G forces

...aerobatics effects, 72-28, 82-13
...simulation with lower body pressure box, 79-8, 82-3, 82-4
...tolerance after crash diet, 81-2
...tolerance effects of antihistamine-decongestant preparations, 78-20

Galactic cosmic radiation

...effect on air carrier crewmembers, 80-2, 92-2, 00-33, 03-16, 05-14

Global positioning system (GPS)

...design considerations, 98-9, 98-12, 99-13, 99-26, 00-4
...effectiveness, 03-17

Handicapped persons

...blind passengers, 80-12
...pilot positions in radar training, 80-5

Heat

...altitude effects on performance, 71-17
...complex performance effects, 69-10, 72-17
...dogs shipped by air transport, 77-8, 81-11, 84-5, 87-8
...human tolerances, 70-22, 71-4
...maintenance of thermal balance, 66-23
...manual performance effects, 68-13
...measurement of evaporative water loss, 63-25
...tolerance limits for rats and mice, 86-8
...tranquilizer effects on loss and conservation, 63-23, 66-14

Hearing

...acoustic signals for emergency evacuation, 79-5
...auditory fatigue, 63-19, 65-1, 65-2
...binaural beat perception, 63-17
...cockpit noise intensities, 68-21, 68-25
...conservation with earplugs, 73-20, 75-11
...earphone transient response, 63-7
...engine noise effects, pilots vs. non-pilots, 05-12
...headset interference tones, 92-4
...interaural intensity difference limen, 67-10
...noise audiometry, 71-1
...noise effects on aircrew personnel, 72-32
...pilots vs. non-pilots, 95-12
...speech intelligibility improvement, 70-6, 72-31, 73-13, 76-3
...table of intensity increments, 66-4
...temporary threshold shift, 79-16, 92-4

Hijacking

...deterrence, 78-35

History (CARI/CAMI)

...historical vignettes, prefaces to 87-1, 97-1, 98-1, 01-1, 03-1, 05-1
...history of aeromedical research contributions, 05-3

Human

...adult female anthropometry, 83-16
...angle of shoulder slope, 65-14
...body center of gravity, 62-14
...body kinematics on deceleration, 62-13
...center of gravity, 62-14, 65-23, 69-22
...child body models, 76-9
...DNA profiling, 98-18
...head injury criteria (HIC) component test device, evaluation, 04-18
...mass distribution of children, 76-9
...pelvis spatial geometry, 82-9
...physical fitness testing, 63-6
...responses to hyperpyrexia, 64-8
...survivability of free-fall impacts, 63-15, 65-12, 68-19
...thorax, determination of effective mass, 96-7
...tolerances, 62-6, 71-3, 71-4, 71-13, 81-2, 82-3, 82-4, 82-10
...tolerances to facial impact, 65-20, 66-12, 66-40
...tolerances to heat, 70-22, 71-4

Human factors (also see: Performance)

...accident reporting system — Human Factors Analysis and Classification System, 00-7, 00-28, 01-3, 03-4, 05-24, 05-25, 06-7, 06-24
...air traffic control operational errors/deviations, role of shiftwork and fatigue, 99-2
  –development of temporal markers to profile, 06-20
  –review of human factors literature, 06-21
  –role of age, 05-22
  –severity index, 05-5
  –evaluation of HFACS and other models to describe causes 05-25
  –strategies for reducing causal factors, 03-19, 06-20
...air traffic sector complexity, 00-24, 03-8, 05-16, 06-29
  –and operational errors, 98-14, 06-4
...Air Traffic Selection and Training (AT-SAT) simulation, 00-2, 00-12
...assessment of complex performance, 69-6, 69-16
...attitude indicators, equivalence tests, 05-23
...auditory startle responses, 88-4
...aviation maintenance, 89-9, 90-14, 91-16, 92-3, 93-5, 93-15, 94-12, 95-14, 95-31, 96-2, 05-21
...aviation safety, 63-35, 66-8, 66-25, 66-27, 70-18, 71-9, 71-10, 72-2, 73-5, 80-6, 92-3, 94-5, 94-27, 99-7, 00-7, 00-28, 01-3, 03-4 04-24, 05-7, 05-15, 05-24, 05-25, 06-7, 06-8, 06-18, 06-26
...CDTI/ADS-B operational evaluation, 00-30, 03-2, 03-5, 03-13, 04-11, 04-20
...color displays and color defect, 06-2, 06-6, 06-11, 06-15, 06-22
...crew resource management, FAA aircrews, 96-24
...decision making, preflight, 96-19, 97-3, 97-23, 98-7, 05-7, 05-15
...emergency evacuation, 65-7, 70-16, 95-25, 96-18, 94-11, 97-20, 98-19, 99-10, 99-30, 03-15
  –FAIT analysis, applied to traffic awareness in free-flight, 03-5
...flight-control problems in unmanned aircraft accident, 06-8
...flight progress strips, 95-4, 95-9, 96-5, 98-26, 00-5
...flight simulator research, 96-15, 96-16, 97-9, 97-24, 98-12, 98-28, 04-20
...GPS use, 98-9, 98-12, 99-9, 99-13, 99-26, 00-4, 03-17
...hearing thresholds of pilots and cockpit warning signals, 05-12

...Human Factors Analysis and Classification System (HFACS), 00-7, 00-28, 01-3, 03-4, 05-24, 06-24
...human factors review of operational error literature, 06-21
...intervention strategies for aircraft accident prevention, 06-24
...JANUS technique applied to ATC operational errors, 03-21, 06-21
...job task taxonomy, 93-1, 95-16
...NEXRAD display use, 04-5
...operational demonstration of flight inspection aircraft, 95-18
...photic stimulation responses, 66-39
...rotorcraft personnel lifting devices, 98-13
...SATORI, 93-12, 97-13, 98-14
...severe weather flying, 66-41, 05-15
...situation awareness and performance in air traffic control, 99-3
...target blink amplitude, attention-getting value, 97-10, 99-8
...unmanned aircraft, accident/incident data, 04-24
–flight-control problems, 06-8
...workstation design, flight inspection aircraft, 95-18
...visual displays, methods to assess information and cognitive complexities, 05-4
...WinMine analytic tool applied to accident data, 06-26

Hypothermia

...passengers, 94-10, 95-20
...wheel-well stowaways, 96-25

Hypoxia

...and beta-blocked hypertensives, 92-19
...blood donation effects, 84-4
...civilian training need, 91-13, 03-10
...human tolerance, 62-6, 63-33
...interaction with marihuana, 75-6
...oxygen need, 66-28, 04-3
...performance decrement, 66-10, 66-15, 71-11, 71-17, 97-9
...propranolol effects, 79-10, 80-10
...sickle cell trait susceptibility, 76-15, 78-30, 80-20
...supersonic transport, decompression in, 99-4
...visual field and glaucoma, 91-1
...wheel-well stowaways, 96-25

Identification

...DNA, profiling of accident victims, 98-18, 99-14
–identification of forensic postmortem specimens, 06-14
...enantiomeric compositions of compounds in cold remedies, 05-8
...sex and race diagnosis from cranial measurements, 79-2

In-flight health care

...medical emergencies, 97-2, 00-13
...medical kits, 91-2, 91-3, 97-2, 00-13

Illusions

...spiral aftereffect, 64-9, 64-10, 64-17, 68-10, 69-15, 71-31
...visual, 70-2, 71-22, 77-12

Injuries

...agricultural aircraft accidents, 72-15, 80-3
...analysis in railroad accident, 73-1
...brain tolerances to concussion, 71-13, 74-4
...cabin safety data bank, 79-23, 82-8
...cockpit delethalization, 66-3, 66-12, 71-3, 72-7, 81-10, 82-7
...correlation with kinematic behavior, 62-13
...criteria for aircraft crashworthiness, 96-11
...decompression of small aircraft, 67-14
...emergency and precautionary evacuations, 79-6, 79-23, 82-8, 99-30, 00-11, 03-15
...eye, 62-12
...facial tolerances to impacts, 65-20
...head impacts while wearing restraint systems, 72-6, 92-20
...head injury criteria (HIC) component test device, evaluation, 04-18
...impact in pregnancy, 68-6, 68-24
...in free falls, 63-15
...neck, 93-14
...padding for crash protection, 66-40
...precautionary evacuations, 99-30
...prevention in aircraft accidents, 71-3, 94-19
...produced by restraint systems, 69-5, 89-3
...rearward-facing seats, 62-7, 69-13
...restraint systems to prevent, 67-13, 69-3, 69-4, 69-5, 69-13, 72-3, 82-7, 83-8, 98-11
...seat impacts, 66-18
...side-facing seats, 69-13
...smoke and fire, 62-9, 70-16
...vertical crash forces, 62-1
...vertical impact in seated position, 62-19
...water impacts, 65-12, 68-19

Instruments

...attitude indicators, 73-9, 05-23
...automation design, measures of information complexity, 04-17
...cockpit displays of traffic information (CDTI), 00-30, 03-2, 03-5, 03-13, 04-11, 04-20
...compact display, effects on performance, 75-12
...GPS, design considerations, 98-9, 98-12, 99-26, 00-4
–effectiveness, 03-17

...head-up displays, 98-28
...Highway-in-the Sky (HITS) displays, 00-31
...NEXRAD weather display, 04-5
...information priorities, 00-26
...navigational display formats, 96-16, 00-8, 04-20
...radiation detection, 71-26
...readability by senior pilots, 77-2, 77-7

Job attitudes

...air traffic controllers, 74-7, 74-12, 75-3, 79-11, 91-10, 00-17, 04-23
...Airway Facilities Service, 77-21, 79-11, 83-7
...aviation business operators, 87-4
...burnout, 92-7
...diversity training, 95-10
...empowerment, perceptions of, 98-24
...exchange ideology, 91-11
...FAA survey 2000, process feedback, 03-11
...FAA survey 2003, agency-wide work attitudes, 04-22
   –Air Traffic Organization work attitudes, 04-23
   –analysis of employee comments, 05-13
...gender, equity, and satisfaction, 92-9
...goal congruence, 92-8
...intent to leave job, 91-15, 06-30
...neuropsychological screening of airmen, 92-11
...organizational change, and cynicism, 99-27, 00-14
...organizational communications, and trust, 99-25
...organizational politics, perceptions of, 92-10
...participation in decision-making, 92-17
...safety behavior, 97-8
...safety perceptions, 99-19
...turnover, and intent to leave job, 91-15, 06-30

Judgment

...decision-making in pilots, 97-3, 97-23, 98-7
...training in pilots, 87-6, 98-6

Kidney

...autoregulation mechanism, 63-32
...effects of acute arterial occlusion, 63-22, 65-27
...effects of increased venous pressure, 62-18, 63-1
...effects of pesticides, 63-26, 66-11

Lighting

...cabin, 79-22, 80-13, 81-7, 98-2
...cockpit, 77-2, 77-13, 77-14, 78-17

Management

...crew resource, FAA flight crews, 96-24
...empowerment, predictors of perceived, 98-24
...ergonometric interventions to reduce worker stress, 99-17
...FAA employee attitude survey, year 2000, process feedback, 03-11
   –year 2003 agency-wide work attitudes, 04-22
   –year 2003 Air Traffic Organization work attitudes, 04-23
   –year 2003 analysis of employer comments, 05-12
...health awareness, survey of FAA programs, 00-3
...job task analysis for supervisors, 91-5
...matrix teams, commitment, 93-18
...organizational change, and cynicism, 99-27, 00-14
...organizational commitment, 92-21
...organizational communication, and technology change, 99-25
...training effectiveness, 75-9, 78-32
...training needs, 90-2
...turnover and intent to leave job, 91-15, 06-30
...workplace safety behaviors, influence on, 97-8
   –employee safety perceptions, 99-19

Medical kits

...used in flight, 91-2, 91-3, 97-2, 00-13

Motion sickness

...susceptibility, 76-14
...treatment effects, 81-16, 82-19

Motivation

...airway facilities personnel, 77-21
...factors in ATC work, 71-30, 74-12
...passengers, in aircraft evacuations, 96-18, 03-15, 04-2

Neurology

...alcohol effects on ataxia test battery, 79-9
...alcohol effects on visual functions, 78-2, 79-15
...brain tolerances to concussion, 71-13, 74-4
...central factor in auditory fatigue, 63-19
...chlordimeform toxicity, 77-19
...conditions associated with aviation safety, 81-3
...drug effects on performance, 64-18
...endrin effects, 63-16, 70-11
...in-flight vertigo and unconsciousness, 63-21
...neuropsychological test battery, 92-11, 95-7
...nucleus rotundus, 77-22
...organophosphate insecticide effects, 63-24, 72-29, 73-3, 73-4, 79-15
...photic stimulation, 66-38
...pupillary movement, 65-9, 65-25
...rheoencephalography in cerebrovascular disease detection, 65-4, 67-11
...seizures in flight, 64-6
...spiral aftereffect test, 64-9, 64-10, 64-17, 68-10, 69-15, 71-31
...studies at GCRI, 64-1
...vestibular tests, 75-4

Noise

...aircrew personnel effects, 72-32
...auditory fatigue, 63-19, 65-1, 65-2
...birds, effects on, 62-4
...ear-protector ratings, 73-20, 75-11
...engine, and pilot vs. non-pilot hearing thresholds, 05-12
...intensity in aircraft cockpits, 68-21, 68-25, 95-18
...performance effects of simulated radar task, 79-24, 83-13
...performance impairment, 72-14
...simulated sonic boom effects, 71-29, 72-19, 72-24, 72-35, 73-16, 74-9
...sonic boom startle effects in field study, 73-11
...speech intelligibility improvement, 70-6, 72-31, 73-13, 76-3
...temporary threshold shift, 79-16

Nystagmus

...adaptation effects, 66-37, 67-6, 67-7, 67-12, 67-19, 69-20
...alcohol effects, 71-6, 71-16, 71-20, 71-34, 71-39, 72-34
...antimotion sickness drug effects, 81-16
...arousal effects, 62-17, 63-29
...caloric habituation, 63-14, 64-14, 65-18, 67-2
...dextroamphetamine and secobarbital effects, 73-17
...habituation to rotation, 63-13, 65-24, 68-2
...illumination effects during angular deceleration, 68-28
...optokinetic stimulation, 70-2, 70-10, 71-22
...secondary, elicitation by irrigation, 63-3
...sleep deprivation, during, 86-9
...translations of reports, Tech. Pub. #1, 64-16, 65-17, 66-2
...vertical, 68-2

Orthostatic tolerance

...alcohol effects at altitude, 82-3
...and beta blocked hypertensives, 92-19
...physical exertion effects, 82-4

Oxygen

...equipment studies, 79-13, 80-18, 89-10, 92-18, 92-22, 95-17, 98-27, 00-6, 04-3, 05-18
...flammability of toiletries, 63-27
...need at altitude, 66-28, 97-9
...need for training among civilians, 91-13, 03-10
...system design, 78-9

Oxygen masks

...crew smoke-protective devices, 76-5, 78-4, 78-14, 78-41, 83-14, 89-8, 89-11, 05-18
...design for children, 66-9
...disposable, 66-7
...donning time after decompression, 66-10
...evaluation, 62-21, 66-7, 66-20, 67-3, 67-9, 72-10, 78-4, 79-13, 80-18, 83-10, 85-10, 87-5, 89-5, 93-6, 96-4, 98-27, 00-6, 04-3, 05-18

Ozone

...chronic effects, 80-16
...effects under simulated flight conditions, 79-20, 80-9
...review of effects, 89-13

Passengers

...aerospace, commercial, guidance for medical screening, 06-1
...blind, cane use in emergency evacuation, 80-12
...child restraints, 94-19, 95-30
...cold/wet exposure, 94-10, 98-4
...commercial aerospace, guidance for medical screening, 06-1
...emergency evacuation, computer model, 72-30, 78-23, 94-11, 97-20
 –experimental cabin, 97-18, 03-15, 04-2
 –infants, 01-18, 05-2
 –precautionary, 99-30, 00-11
 –seating configurations, 89-14, 03-15
 –size of exits, 99-10
...emergency lighting, floor, 98-2
...flow rates between compartments, 78-3
...handicapped emergency evacuation, 77-11, 80-12
...head injury analysis, 92-20
...human external loads, rotorcraft, 98-13
...illness and injuries, cabin safety data bank, 79-23
...injuries, during emergency evacuation, 79-6, 79-23, 03-15
 –during precautionary evacuation, 99-30
...medical kits, use of, 91-2, 91-3
...neck injury analysis, 93-14
...oxygen masks, 79-13, 80-18, 95-17, 96-4
...ozone effects, 80-9, 89-13
...protective breathing devices, 67-4, 70-20, 83-10, 85-10, 87-2, 87-5, 89-5, 05-18
...safety information, availability, 04-19
...sport parachutists, 98-11
...water spray exposure, 98-4
...wheel-well stowaways, 96-25

Patients

...air transport with eye injuries, 62-12
...civilian air ambulance services, 71-18, 82-5
...human external loads, 98-13
...supplemental oxygen from Molecular Sieve oxygen concentrators, 92-22

Perception

...anticollision lights, 66-39, 70-9, 70-15, 71-42
...approach angle in simulated night landings, 81-6, 82-6
...auditory fatigue, 63-19
...binaural beat, 63-17
...Broca-Sulzer phenomenon, 68-27
...color, 67-8, 83-11, 90-9, 06-2, 06-6, 06-11, 06-15, 06-22
...depth, 63-10, 63-28, 65-11, 65-32, 67-20, 00-18
...highlighted targets on displays, 97-10, 99-8
...induced decrements, 93-19
...interaural intensity difference limen, 67-10
...matching loudness to flash brightness, 67-16
...peripheral visual cues, 68-11, 68-12, 68-22
...propeller paint schemes, 78-29
...reaction time, flash luminance and brightness, 67-24
...size and distance, 62-15, 64-13, 66-22, 66-24, 67-18
...spatial extent, 63-20
...spiral aftereffect, 64-9, 64-10, 68-10, 69-15, 71-31
...tactile, 62-11, 62-16
...two-flash thresholds, 68-20, 70-15
...vision through sunscreen materials, 78-28

Performance (also see: Human Factors)

...accident experience, physical defects, 76-7, 77-20, 79-19, 81-14, 83-18
...age effects, 95-3, 95-7, 99-20, 99-22
...age index for pilots, 77-6, 78-16, 78-27, 83-15, 85-3
...age 60 rule, 94-20, 94-21, 94-22, 94-23, 04-8
...airspace complexity, 05-16
  –and operational errors, 06-4
...air traffic controllers
  –age and retirement, 05-6, 05-22
  –age effects, 61-1, 62-3, 65-21, 67-1, 71-36, 73-7, 81-12, 84-6, 99-18, 99-23, 05-22
  –aptitude tests for prediction, 65-19, 68-14, 71-28, 71-36, 71-40, 72-18, 79-3, 84-2, 84-6, 88-3, 89-6, 94-4, 97-15, 98-23, 99-16, 00-2, 00-12. 06-16
  –color displays and color defect, 06-2, 06-6, 06-11, 06-15, 06-22
  –color perception effects, 83-11, 90-3
  –communication, ATC/pilot, 93-20, 95-15, 96-10, 96-20, 96-26, 98-17, 98-20, 99-21, 01-8, 01-9, 05-19, 06-25
  –commuter (driving) risk factor before and after shifts, 06-13
  –computer experience and AT-SAT performance, 00-2
  –development of temporal markers to profile, 06-20
  –evaluation, 61-1, 65-22, 98-23
  –experience as predictor, 63-31
  –flight service station training, 86-6
  –flashing target effects, 90-3, 97-10, 99-8
  –human factors literature review, 06-21
  –incident reporting, 65-10
  –information complexity measures in automation design, 04-17
  –information and cognitive complexity assessment methods, 05-4
  –job task taxonomy for en route, 93-1
  –measurement in air traffic selection and training (AT-SAT) simulation, 00-2, 00-12
  –memory in air traffic control, 97-22, 98-16.
  –navigation displays, 00-8, 04-20
  –Multiple Task Performance Battery for selection, 72-5, 74-10
  –napping and night shift performance, 00-10
  –no relation to age, 05-22
  –operational errors, development of temporal markers to profile, 06-20
  –operational errors, human factors literature review, 06-21
  –operational errors, JANUS technique applied to causal factors, 03-21
  –operational errors/deviations, role of shiftwork and fatigue, 99-2
  –pass-fail in FSS training program, 79-18
  –personality factors, relation to, 70-14, 89-7, 03-20, 04-21
  –radar simulator, 65-31, 75-8, 77-18, 78-11, 80-15, 80-17, 82-1, 82-16, 83-9, 83-13, 86-4, 88-4, 89-1, 90-3, 95-23
  –sector characteristics, activity and complexity, 06-29
  –sector characteristics and operational errors, 87-15, 06-4
  –sex differences, 72-22
  –situation awareness, 94-27, 98-16, 99-3
  –strategies for reducing causal factors, 03-19
  –video game experience as a predictor, 97-4
...airworthiness inspectors, 87-4
...alcohol effects, 66-29, 69-14, 71-20, 71-34, 72-4, 72-11, 72-34, 78-2, 79-7, 79-26, 82-3, 83-2, 85-5, 88-2, 94-24, 95-3, 95-7, 95-24
...antihistamine effects, at altitude, 68-15, 78-19
  –on performance, 97-25, 99-20
...attitude indicators (flight instrument), 73-9, 05-23
...attitude questionnaires to predict under stress, 69-7
...aural glide slope cues for instrument approaches, 71-24
...aviation medical examiners, 84-7
...chronic disulfoton poisoning effects, 69-19
...cockpit instrument display, compact, 75-12

–Cockpit Display of Traffic Information (CDTI), 03-2, 03-5, 03-13, 04-11, 04-20
–Electronic Attitude Direction Indicator (EADI), equivalence tests, 05-23
–GPS, 98-9, 98-12, 99-9, 99-13, 00-4, 03-19
–head-up, 98-28
–Highway-in-the-Sky (HITS), 00-31
–NEXRAD weather, 04-5
...cognitive appraisal of stress effects, 68-17
...cognitive style and learning, 99-12
...crash diet effects, 81-8
...decompression effects, 66-10
...dextroamphetamine effects during sleep loss, 75-14
...distractibility effects, 72-25
...distracting stimuli effects, 71-7, 72-14
...drug effects, during angular acceleration, 73-17, 82-19
–in aircraft simulator, 64-18
–on complex performance, 69-9, 75-14, 77-17, 78-19, 97-25, 99-20
...eye blink-rate measures, 94-17, 94-26, 96-9, 99-28
...flight instructors and accidents, 96-3
...flight simulation, 96-16, 97-9, 97-24, 98-12, 04-5, 05-23
...forest fire retardant missions, effects of, 68-26
...gender effects and antihistamine, 99-20
...heart disease and age effects, 64-4
...heat and altitude effects, 71-17
...heat effects on complex performance, 69-10, 72-17
...Human Factors Analysis and Classification System (HFACS), 00-7, 00-28, 01-3, 03-4, 05-24, 05-25, 06-7, 06-18, 06-24
...human factors, review of operational errors literature, 06-21
...hypoxia, decrement due to, 66-15, 71-11, 82-10, 83-15, 85-3, 85-5, 97-9
...impairment by alcohol, 66-29, 69-14, 71-20, 71-34, 72-4, 72-11, 72-34, 78-2, 79-7, 79-26, 82-3, 83-2, 85-5, 88-2, 94-24, 95-3, 95-7, 95-24
...instrument flying using peripheral visual cues, 68-11, 68-12, 68-22
...intercontinental flight effects, 65-16, 65-28, 65-29, 65-30, 68-8, 69-17
...laser illumination effects on flight simulator performance, 03-12, 04-9
...marihuana effects, 73-12, 75-6, 85-8
...measurement, 77-15, 78-33, 78-34, 84-2, 98-23, 99-22, 00-2, 00-5, 05-23
...mental task effects on auditory fatigue, 65-1, 65-2
...monotonous task correlates, 73-14, 75-8
...noise effects on simulated radar task, 79-24
...Phosdrin effects, 72-29, 73-3
...physical conditioning program effects, 66-17, 66-21

...physical exercise effects, 82-4, 82-10
...physiological measures, on perceptual-motor tasks, 69-8
–in severe weather flying, 66-41
...pilot tracking during successive approaches, 72-9
...pseudopilots in radar training, 80-5
...psychophysiological indices, 99-28
...readiness to perform, 93-13, 95-24, 97-5
...reliability of individual subjects, 78-37
...rotating shifts, 96-23, 99-2
–and commuting risk factors before and after shifts, 06-13
...shifts in wake-sleep cycle, effects, 75-10, 76-11
...signal rate effects on monitoring, 69-6, 69-16, 97-10
...simulated autopilot malfunctions, 97-24
...simulated glidepath indicators, 79-4, 79-25, 81-6, 82-6
...situation assessment through re-creation of incidents (SATORI), 93-12, 97-13, 98-14
...situation awareness, effects, 99-3, 00-31
–FAIT analysis for free-flight environment, 03-5
...sleep deprivation, effects, 70-8, 85-3
–quality and ATC performance, 00-10
...smoking effects, 80-11, 83-4, 97-7
...sonic boom effects, 71-29, 72-19, 74-9
...startle effects, 69-21, 73-11, 73-16, 79-24, 83-13, 88-4
...stress-related decrements, 93-19
...student pilots, 67-15, 69-12
...tasks for operator-skills research, 66-19
...teamwork training, 99-24
...time-sharing ability, 76-1, 99-22
...tracking and complex performance, 72-21
...tracking, dextroamphetamine, sleep loss, 76-12
...video game experience, on ATC selection tests, 97-4
...visual search with and without radar sweepline, 79-12
...visual taskload effects on CFF change during complex monitoring, 85-13
...visual taskload effects on complex monitoring, 88-1, 90-3, 95-23
...weather information (NEXRAD) and simulator performance, 04-5
...work in heat and cold, 66-23, 68-13

Personnel, FAA (see also, Air Traffic Controllers)

...airway facilities personnel, job attitudes, 77-21, 79-11, 83-7
...Airway Science Curriculum Demonstration Project, evaluation of, 88-5
...airworthiness inspectors, job performance ratings of, 87-4

Part III: Subject Index

...biological rhythms and rotating shiftwork considerations, 86-2
...correlates of satisfaction with training, 91-9
...decision making, equity, and job satisfaction, 91-10
...effectiveness of management training, 75-9, 78-32, 92-16
...electronics technicians, 97-19
...employee attitude survey, year 2000, process feedback, 03-11
  –year 2003 agency-wide work attitudes, 04-22
  –year 2003 Air Traffic Organization work attitudes, 04-23
  –year 2003 analysis of employee comments, 05-12
...empowerment, predictors of perceived, 98-24
...ergonomic interventions to reduce work stress, 99-17
...flight inspection aircrews, crew resource management, 96-24
...flight service station, organizational climate, 97-12
...health awareness programs, survey evaluation, 00-3
...intent to leave job, and active turnover, 06-30
  –job satisfaction, 91-15
...identification of management training needs, 90-2, 92-16
...identification with occupation, 92-21
...job task analysis for FAA supervisors, 91-5
...job task taxonomy, en route, 93-1
...maintenance, 89-9, 90-14, 91-16, 92-3, 93-5, 93-15, 94-12, 95-14, 95-31, 96-2, 05-21
...matrix teams, 93-18
...organizational change, and cynicism, 99-27, 00-14
...organizational commitment, 92-21
...organizational communication, and technology change, 99-25
...organizational support, perceptions of, 92-13
...safety perceptions following safety awareness program, 99-19
...team implementation and diversity climate, 00-27
...test fairness for selection, 79-3, 96-13, 99-16

Pesticides

...aerial application aircraft accidents, 66-27, 66-30, 68-16, 78-31, 80-3
...biochemical effects of lindane and dieldrin, 62-10, 63-4
...chlordimeform toxicity, 77-19
...cholinesterase determination, 67-5
...CNS, effects of organophosphates, 63-24, 69-19, 79-15
...comparison of serum cholinesterase methods, 70-13, 72-12
...dieldrin effects on liver, 66-5, 66-26
...endrin effects, 66-11, 66-26, 66-34, 70-11
...endrin, mechanisms of action, 63-16, 63-26
...methamidophos toxicity, 78-26
...organophosphates effects on reproduction, 70-3
...Phosdrin effects on performance, 72-29, 73-3
...Phosdrin effects on vision, 73-4
...storage stability of human blood cholinesterase, 70-4
...symptoms and treatment of poisoning, 62-8

Physical fitness

...aerospace, commercial passengers, guidance for medical screening, 06-1
...age relationship, 63-18
...ATC students, 71-8
...field test for, 63-6
...myocardial infarction, 64-2, 66-17, 66-21
...neuropsychological screening, 92-11

Physiology

...autonomic and performance, 93-19
...backscatter, responses to, 72-8
...blood donation effects, 84-4
...cabin water spray, following, 98-4
...crash diet effects, 81-2, 81-8
...evaporative water loss device, 67-17
...gas pressure in tissue, 63-11
...high altitude training, need for, 91-13
...hydrogen ion concentration, conversion table from pH, 68-23
...measures during complex task performance, 69-8, 82-10
...neural control of the ciliary muscle, 63-5
...protection at high altitude, 99-4
...sleep deprivation responses, 70-8, 75-14
...smoking withdrawal responses, 83-4
...thermal balance, 66-23
...tolerances to heat, 70-22, 71-4
...wheel-well stowaways, 96-25

Pilots

...accident experience, physical defects, 76-7, 77-20, 79-19, 81-14, 83-18
...accident predisposition, 72-2, 73-5
  –organizational factors, 00-28
...active population, estimate of, 68-5
...aerial applicator protection, 66-30, 72-15, 80-3
...age index, 77-6, 78-16, 78-27, 82-18
...age 60 rule, 94-20, 94-21, 94-22, 94-23, 04-8
...ages of those in aircraft accidents, 67-22, 70-18, 77-10, 94-22
...alcohol effects on performance, 66-29, 72-4, 79-7, 79-26
...alcoholic airline pilots rehabilitation, 85-12
...altitude tolerance with pulmonary disease, 77-16

...analysis of certification denial actions, 68-9, 74-5, 76-10, 78-25, 80-19, 83-5, 84-9, 85-9, 86-7, 90-5, 90-7
...anticollision observing responses, 73-6
...attitudes toward safety, 95-27, 05-7
 –toward safety training, 97-16, 98-6, 99-7, 03-10
...attrition, 72-13, 73-8
...blood donation effects, 84-4
...blood pressure levels, 84-3
...cardiovascular health changes in third-class certificate holders, 72-26
...Cockpit Display of Traffic Information (CDTI), FIAT, 03-5, 03-13, 04-11, 04-20
...cockpit visual problems, 77-2, 77-7, 77-13, 77-14, 78-17, 03-12
...color vision and signal lights, 71-27, 71-32, 73-18, 75-1, 93-17
...communication, 96-10, 96-20, 96-26, 98-17, 98-20, 99-21, 06-25
...computer-based flight simulator, 96-15
...computer use, in meeting recency of experience flight requirements, 03-3
 –in flight training, 94-25, 95-6, 96-8, 97-11
...control force capabilities of females, 72-27, 73-23
...coronary atherosclerosis in fatal accidents, 80-8, 85-6
...crew resource management, flight inspection aircrew, 96-24
...decision-making skills, 98-7
...decision-making training, 87-6, 96-19, 98-6
 –"expert" pilot training model, 97-6
 –use of weather information, 97-3, 97-23, 04-5, 05-7, 05-15
...demographics and vision restrictions, 04-6
...disease prevalence and incidence, 73-8, 81-9, 84-8, 89-2
...drug effects in aircraft simulator, 64-18
...engine noise and hearing thresholds, 05-12
...exams of first-class certificate holders by senior AMEs, 71-38
...experience in controller selection, 74-8
...fatigue, 81-13
...flight information accessed by pilots, 00-26
...flight physiology training, need for, 91-13, 03-10
...G effects of aerobatics, 72-28, 82-13
...glare exposure and accidents, 03-6, 06-28
...hearing, vs. non-pilots, 05-12
...heart rates during instrument approaches, 70-7, 71-24, 75-12
...heat effects on performance in a flight simulator, 72-17
...judgment training, 87-6
...laser light illumination incidents, 06-23
...longevity and survival of retired airline pilots, 95-5

...marginal weather and willingness to take off, 05-7, 05-15
...marijuana in general aviation fatal accidents, 85-8
...medical standards, 71-25, 82-14
...medications found postmortem and medical history, 06-12
...navigation displays, moving map, 04-20
 –using text and graphics, 00-8
...neuropsychological screening, 92-11
...noise effects on hearing, 72-32, 05-12
...occupations, 69-11, 77-10
...ozone effects, 80-9, 89-13
...performance, on glidepath indicator systems, 79-4, 79-25, 81-6, 82-6
 –electronic attitude-direction indicator (EADI), 05-23
 –GPS displays, 98-9, 98-12, 99-9, 99-13, 99-26, 03-17
 –head-up displays, 98-28
 –Highway-in-the Sky (HITS) display, 00-31
 –NEXRAD weather display, 04-5
 –simulated autopilot malfunctions, 97-24
 –two attitude indicators, 73-9
...peripheral visual cue response, 68-11, 68-12, 68-22
...physician accidents, 66-25, 71-9
...physiological responses on cross-country flights, 71-23
...physiological studies in air tankers, 68-26
...pulmonary function, 77-3
...risk factors for cardiac events, 90-7
...safety climate, pilot perception of, 00-28
...safety training, evaluation, 97-16, 98-6, 99-7, 03-10
...satisfaction with ATC services, 90-6
...severe weather flying, 66-41, 05-7, 05-15
...shoulder harness, use of, 95-2
...smoking effects on performance, 80-11, 83-4
...status variables with accidents, 70-18
...stress, domestic-based and perceived performance, 00-32
...stress in student pilots, 67-15, 69-12, 76-2
...suicide, 72-2, 73-5, 06-5
...tracking performance during successive approaches, 72-9
...type airman certificate related to accidents, 67-23
...vertigo, 67-19
...visual acuity, midair collisions, 75-5
...voice communication, 93-20, 06-25
...workload, 77-15, 81-13

Pregnancy

...crewmember radiation exposure, 92-2, 00-33, 03-16
...emergency air transport, 82-5

...impact injuries, 68-6, 68-24
...organophosphate pesticide effects in rats, 70-3

Propellers

...paint schemes conspicuity, 78-29
...propeller-to-person accidents, 81-15, 93-2

Protective breathing equipment

...evaluation, 62-21, 66-7, 66-20, 67-3, 67-9, 72-10, 78-4, 79-13, 80-18, 83-10, 85-10, 87-5, 89-5, 93-6, 96-4, 98-27, 00-6, 04-3, 05-18

Psychology

...accident proneness, 93-9
...air traffic controllers and retirement age, 05-6, 05-22
...aircraft mix and traffic complexity ratings, 05-16
...automation and pilot performance, 97-24, 00-8
...CogScreen, neuropsychological test, age effects, 99-22
...cognitive complexity in an air traffic control displays, 05-4
...cognitive style and learning, 99-12
...Composite Mood Adjective Check List to measure stress effects, 71-14, 71-21, 73-22
...cultural diversity awareness training, 95-10
...disability retirement, and ATC personality factors, 03-14
...diversity climate, 00-26
...empowerment, predictors of perceived, 98-24
...expertise method in aeronautical decision- making, 97-6
...FAA employee attitude survey, year 2000, process feedback, 03-11
 –year 2003 agency-wide work attitudes, 04-22
 –year 2003 Air Traffic Organization work attitudes, 04-23
 –year 2003 analysis of employee comments, 05-12
...flight inspection aircraft, preferences, 95-18
...Human Factors Analysis and Classification System (HFACS) applications, 00-7, 00-28, 01-3, 03-4, 05-24, 05-25, 06-7, 06-18, 06-24
...human factors review of operational error literature, 06-21
...JANUS technique and causal factors in ATC operational errors, 03-21
...job attitudes, airway facilities personnel, 77-21, 79-11, 83-7
...memory in air traffic control, 97-22, 98-16
...motivation in aircraft evacuation, 96-18, 03-15, 04-2
...Myers-Briggs personality test with ATCSs, 04-21

...organizational factors, 90-2, 91-5, 92-8, 92-9, 92-10, 92-13, 92-17, 92-21, 05-1294-2, 98-23, 99-25, 99-27, 00-14, 00-27, 03-11, 04-22, 04-23, 05-12
...personality assessment, 71-35, 91-8, 93-4, 03-14, 04-21
...pilot attitudes toward safety, 95-27, 98-7, 99-7, 05-7, 05-15
...psychological autopsy, 72-2, 73-5
...psychophysiological indices of alertness, 99-28
...safety behaviors on the job, management influence, 97-8, 99-19
...Shipley Institute of Living Scale with ATCSs, 92-30
...situational awareness, 94-27, 97-13, 97-22, 98-16, 99-3, 00-31, 03-5, 03-13
...Sixteen Personality Factors test with ATCSs, 97-17, 03-14
...stress and anxiety in air traffic controllers, 80-14, 81-5, 89-7
...stress, domestic-based and perceived pilot performance, 00-32
 –physical symptoms in employees, 99-17
...Type A behavior, 86-4, 94-13
...use of PC-based training devices, 94-25, 95-6, 96-8, 96-15, 96-16, 97-11, 03-3
...validity coefficients in ATCS selection, 00-15

Pulmonary

...disease, altitude tolerance, 77-16
...function testing, 64-1, 71-8, 77-3
...glyceryl trinitrate, vascular effects of, 64-11
...hyperpyrexia, responses to, 64-8
...ozone effects on function, 79-20, 80-9, 89-13
...protection from smoke, fire, 67-4, 78-4, 83-10, 83-14, 85-10
...thromboembolism, 64-7

Radiation

...calibration of Concorde detection instrument, 71-26
...cosmic, and air carrier crewmembers, 92-2, 00-33, 03-16, 05-14
...measurements at SST altitudes, 71-26, 80-2
...RBE of fast neutrons, 78-8
...transport limits for radioactive material, 82-12

Renal function

...acute arterial occlusion effects, 63-22, 65-27
...autoregulation mechanism, 63-32
...insecticide effects, 63-26
...venous pressure effects, increase of, 62-18, 63-1

Research, aeromedical

...aging studies at GCRI, 64-1
...aims and accomplishments, 62-20, 67-25
...alcohol effects review, low dose, 94-24
...ballistocardiography, 64-12, 65-8, 65-15
...beta blockers, analysis and differentiation, 04-15, 05-10
...bibliography of acceleration studies, 63-30
...bibliography of shiftwork research, 83-17
...butalbital, distribution of fluids and tissues, 00-29
...carboxyhemoglobin standard, 98-21
...color vision, 67-8, 71-27, 71-32, 73-18, 75-1, 83-11, 85-7, 92-6, 92-28, 92-29, 93-16, 93-17, 95-13, 96-22, 04-10, 04-14, 06-2, 06-6, 06-11, 06-15, 06-22
...commuting risk factors, before and after work shifts, 06-13
...DNA, detection of postmortem ethanol-producing microorganisms, 00-16
 –identification of forensic samples, 06-14
...DNA profiling, 98-18, 99-14, 06-14
...enantiomeric analysis of ephedrines and norephedrines, 05-8
...exercise, 64-2, 66-36
...hearing, conservation with earplugs, 73-20, 75-11
...history, CAMI, prefaces to 87-1, 97-1, 98-1, 01-1, 03-1, 05-1
 –CAMI research contributions from 1,000 technical reports, 05-3
...index of international publications, 93-3
...index of OAM reports, 63-2, 64-20, 66-1, 68-1, 70-1, 72-1, 74-1, 77-1, 79-1, 81-1, 83-1, 87-1, 90-1, 92-1, 94-1, 96-1, 97-1, 98-1, 99-1, 00-1, 01-1, 03-1, 05-1
...interpretation of carboxyhemoglobin and cyanide concentrations, 05-9
...medical care, inflight, 00-13
...medical incapacitation and impairment of pilots inflight, 04-16
...medical incidents inflight, 00-13
...needs, 63-35, 71-10
...noise effects on aircrew personnel, 72-32
...opiates vs. poppy seed use, postmortem determinations, 05-11
...postmortem, cocaine analysis, 03-23, 03-24
 –accurate assignment of ethanol origin, 04-13
 –ethanol analysis, internal standard, 98-5
 –identification of forensic specimens, 06-14
...plans, for NAS operator selection, 97-19
...radiation, galactic, 92-2, 00-33, 03-16, 05-14
...RNA isolation from peripheral blood cells, protocol validation, 04-1
...quinine elimination, 94-16

...stain test for dieldrin and endrin, 66-26
...translated material, Tech. Pub. #1, 64-16, 65-17, 66-2, 68-7, 71-5, 76-4, 81-4
...visual standards and tests used with aircraft maintenance personnel, 05-21

Restraint

...acceptance of upper torso restraint, 71-12
...bibliography, 63-30
...center of gravity, 62-14, 65-23, 69-22
...child, 94-19, 95-30
...cockpit delethalization, 66-3, 71-3, 72-6, 81-10
...comparison of systems, 67-13, 69-3, 69-4, 69-5, 69-13
...effectiveness in agricultural aircraft accidents, 72-15, 80-3
...evaluation, 78-6, 78-24, 79-17
...head impacts while wearing, 72-6
...infant and child systems, 78-12
...kinematics with seatbelt restraint, 62-13, 92-20
...lapbelt effects on pregnant female, 68-24
...push-button buckles, 99-6
...shoulder harness benefits, 72-3, 82-7, 83-8
...shoulder harness design, 65-14
...sport parachutists, 98-11
...upper body restraint installation, 66-33

Seat

...child and infant seat evaluation, 78-12, 94-19, 95-30
...comfort, 62-1
...cushion flotation, 66-13, 95-20
...energy-absorbing, 83-3, 90-11
...evaluation, 78-6, 78-24, 79-17, 80-3, 81-10, 82-7, 83-3
...fire-blocking materials toxicity, 86-1
...head injury criteria (HIC) component test device, evaluation, 04-18
...injury potential, 66-18, 71-3, 72-15, 82-7, 83-8, 89-3
...pitch and evacuation, 92-27
...placement and Type III exits, 95-22
...pressure distribution, 62-1
...rearward-facing, injuries, 62-7, 69-13
...side-facing, impact injuries, 69-13

Seatbelts

...center of gravity in design, 62-14, 65-23
...cockpit delethalization, 66-3, 71-3
...evaluation of different systems, 67-13, 69-3, 69-13
...impact injuries due to, 69-5
...impact injuries to pregnant females, 68-24
...kinematics of restrained subjects, 62-13
...push-button buckles, 99-6

Shiftwork and shift rotations

...attitudes of ATCSs, 73-2
...bibliography of shiftwork research, 83-17
...commuting risk factors before and after shifts, 06-13
...8- vs. 10-hour work schedules, 95-32
...5-day and 2-2-1 pattern, 73-22, 75-7, 95-12, 95-19, 96-23
...performance effects, shifts and antihistamines, 97-25
  –shifts and fatigue, 99-2
...review, 86-2
...sleep in air traffic controllers, 77-5, 95-12, 95-19, 99-2, 00-10
...steady and 2-2-1 shifts, 85-2
...symptoms reported for ATCSs, 65-5, 65-6
...translations of reports, 81-4

Shoulder harness

...acceptance tests, 71-12
...angle of shoulder slope in design, 65-14
...benefits, 72-3, 82-7, 83-8
...cockpit delethalization, 66-3, 72-6, 81-10
...comparison of types, 67-13, 69-3, 69-4, 69-5
...effectiveness in agricultural aircraft accidents, 72-15, 80-3
...failures, 81-10
...head impacts while wearing, 72-6
...installation in general aviation aircraft, 66-33
...use of, 95-2

Sickle cell trait

...aeromedical significance, 76-15, 80-20
...research protocol, 78-30

Simulation

...advanced general aviation cockpit displays for visual flight procedures, 04-20, 05-23
...air traffic controller radar task, 65-31, 75-8, 77-18, 78-11, 79-12, 79-24, 80-15, 81-12, 82-1, 82-16, 83-9, 83-13, 90-3, 94-17, 94-26, 96-9, 99-3, 00-2, 00-5
...air traffic controller color perception and job performance, 83-11, 90-9, 92-6
...Air Traffic Selection and Training (AT-SAT), 00-2
  –and personality test scores, 03-20
...aircraft passenger emergency evacuation, 72-30, 77-11, 78-23, 96-18, 97-18, 00-15, 04-2, 04-12
...approach control and communication, 98-17
...autopilot malfunctions and pilot responses, 97-24
...aviation stress protocol, 78-5
...electronic attitude direction indicator, PFD equivalency, 05-23
...flight, PC-based, 96-15, 96-16
  –and performance, 97-9

...GPS displays, 98-9, 98-12
...head-up displays, 98-28
...Highway-in-the Sky (HITS) display, 00-31
...+Gz, 79-8
...laser illumination effects on pilot responses, 03-12, 04-9
...movement of objects in depth, 65-32
...navigation display formats, 96-16
...NEXRAD weather displays and flight performance, 04-5
...night approaches to landing, 77-12, 78-15, 79-4, 81-6, 82-6
...operator skills research, 66-19
...pilot workload, 77-15, 82-10, 83-15
...sonic booms, 71-29, 72-19, 72-24, 72-35, 73-16
...stress in ground trainer use, 76-2
...transfer of training, 69-24
...visual glidepath indicator systems, 79-4, 79-25, 81-6, 82-6

Skin

...conductance with sonic booms, 71-29
...evaporative water loss, 63-25
...flammability of toiletries, 63-27
...galvanic skin response, 64-18
...tactile communication, 62-11, 62-16
...temperature to predict tolerances to heat and cold, 71-4
...thermal stress following cabin water spray, 98-4

Sleep

...air traffic controllers, 77-5, 95-12, 95-19, 00-10, 06-13
...deprivation, 70-8, 85-3
...dextroamphetamine effects during sleep loss, 75-14
...loss, and performance, 93-19
  –and vestibular response, 86-9
...shiftwork effects in sleep-wake cycle, 75-10, 76-11
...sonic boom effects, 72-19, 72-24, 72-35
...work schedule effects, 95-32, 99-2, 00-10

Smoke

...air carrier accidents, 62-9, 65-7, 70-16
...crew protective devices, 76-5, 78-4, 78-14, 78-41, 83-14, 89-8, 89-11
...emergency signs, effects on reading, 79-22, 80-13, 81-7
...passenger protective breathing devices, 67-4, 70-20, 83-10, 85-10, 87-2, 87-5, 89-5, 89-12, 05-18
...toxicity, 95-8
...toxicity of thermal degradation products of engine oils, 83-12

Smoking

...aviation safety, effects on, 80-11, 97-7
...smoking/withdrawal effects, 83-4

Sonic booms

...autonomic responses, 71-29, 72-35, 73-16, 74-9
...sleep, effects during, 72-19, 72-24, 72-35
...startle effects, 73-11, 73-16, 74-9
...tracking performance effects, 71-29

Stalls

...warning device, 66-31

Standards

...advanced aerospace systems, 71-33
...aeromedical, 71-25, 71-33, 82-14, 00-19
...carboxyhemoglobin, 98-21
...color vision for air traffic controllers, 83-11, 90-9, 04-10, 04-14, 06-2, 06-6, 06-11, 06-15, 06-22
...escape slides, inflatable, 98-3
...floor proximity marking systems, 98-2
...head injury criteria (HIC) component test device, evaluation, 04-18
...neurological and neurosurgical conditions, 81-3
...postmortem ethanol analysis, internal standard, 98-5
  –accurate assignment of ethanol origin, 04-13
...quality assurance in forensic toxicology, 99-11, 99-15, 03-18, 04-15

Stress

...air tanker pilots, 68-26
...air traffic controllers, 71-2, 71-21, 73-15, 73-21, 73-22, 74-11, 75-7, 76-13, 77-23, 78-5, 78-18, 78-40, 80-14, 82-17, 05-7
...assessment with State-Trait Anxiety Inventory, 72-23, 81-5, 91-8
...aviation stress protocol—simulation, 78-5
...Composite Mood Adjective Check List, to measure, 71-14, 71-21
...domestic-based and pilots' perceived performance, 00-32
...ergonomic interventions, 99-17
...evaporative water loss device, 67-17
...flight inspection crews, 81-13
...+Gz, 79-8
...heart rate and performance effects, 68-17, 69-21
...heart rates during instrument approaches, 70-7, 71-24, 75-12
...job and burnout, 92-7
...measurement of evaporative water loss, 63-25
...monotony with automation as a stressor, 80-1
...performance prediction by attitudes, 69-7
...performance under auditory distraction, 72-14

...physiological responses on cross-country flights, 71-23
...plasma catecholamine determination, 66-6, 71-15
...severe weather flying, 66-41
...situational in accident causation, 72-2, 73-5
...student pilots, 67-15, 69-12, 76-2
...symptoms reported by air traffic controllers, 65-5, 65-6
...urinary metabolites, 78-18, 78-40, 85-2
...wake-sleep cycle shifts, 75-10, 76-11

Suicide

...aircraft accident cause, 72-2, 73-5, 06-5

Supersonic transport

...anticollision lights, 70-9, 70-15, 71-42
...decompression profiles, 70-12, 99-4
...evacuation tests, 70-19
...radiation at SST altitudes, 71-26, 80-2
...sonic boom effects, 71-29, 72-19, 72-24, 72-35, 73-11, 73-16, 74-9

Temperature

...cold effects on shipped dogs, 87-2
...changes in cold water with prototype life preserver, 85-11
...complex performance effects, 69-10, 71-17, 72-17
...evaporative water loss, 63-25, 67-17
...heat effects on shipped dogs, 77-8, 81-11, 84-5, 87-8
...heat tolerance limits of rats and mice, 86-8
...human tolerance, 62-6, 70-22
...hyperpyrexia, 64-8
...liver damage effects by dieldrin, 66-5
...maintenance of thermal balance, 66-23
...manual performance effects, 68-13
...tranquilizer effects on body temperature, 63-23, 66-14

Tests

...air traffic controller selection, 61-1, 62-2, 65-19, 65-21, 68-14, 71-28, 71-36, 72-5, 72-18, 74-10, 77-25, 78-7, 79-3, 79-14, 79-21, 80-7, 82-11, 84-2, 84-6, 90-4, 90-8, 90-13, 91-9, 94-4, 94-9, 96-13, 97-4, 97-15, 98-23, 99-16, 99-23, 00-2, 00-12, 03-20, 06-16
...alcohol abuse, 83-2
...aptitude measures, of military ATCS trainees, 71-40
  –of female ATCS trainees, 72-22
...Armstrong Laboratory Aviation Personality Survey, with ATCS students, 03-20
...ataxia, alcohol effects, 79-9
...ballistocardiography, 64-12, 65-8, 65-15
...cholinesterase activity, 67-5

...color vision, 67-8, 71-27, 71-32, 73-18, 75-1, 83-11, 85-7, 90-9, 92-29, 93-16, 93-17, 95-13, 04-10, 04-14, 06-2
...complex human performance, 69-6, 69-16, 72-5, 72-21
...CogScreen, age effects, 99-22
...Composite Mood Adjective Check List, 71-14, 71-21, 73-22
...correlation with experience in ATCS selection, 63-31
...directional headings, 72-18, 90-8
...distraction susceptibility, 71-7
...emergency evacuation, 65-7, 66-42, 70-19, 70-20, 77-11, 78-3, 79-5, 89-5, 89-14, 92-27, 95-22, 95-25, 96-18, 99-10, 01-18 03-15, 04-2, 05-2
...energy-absorbing seat effectiveness, 83-3, 90-11
...equivalence tests, EADI and PFD displays, 05-23
...escape slides, inflatable, 98-3
...fairness, 79-3, 96-13, 98-23, 99-16
...flight service station training, 79-18, 86-6
...head injury criteria (HIC) component test device, evaluation, 04-18
...interpretation of carboxyheloglobin and cyanide concentration in aviation accidents, 05-9
...Myers-Briggs personality test, with ATCs, 04-21
...NEO Personality Inventory-Revised, with ATCS students, 03-20
...neuropsychological battery, 92-11, 99-22
...performance, 66-19, 97-5, 00-2
 –age and disease, 64-4
 –and age, 65-21, 71-36, 81-12, 99-23
 –and personality factors, 70-14
 –post decompression, 66-10
 –with hypoxia, 66-15, 71-11, 82-10, 83-15
...personality assessment, 71-35, 93-4, 03-20
...physical fitness, 63-6, 63-18, 63-33, 64-3, 66-17
...proficiency in post mortem forensic toxicology, 99-11
...pupillary movement, 65-9, 65-25
...readiness to perform, 93-13, 95-24
...scanning and monitoring, 92-12, 94-8
...Shipley Institute of Living Scale, 92-30
...Sixteen Personality Factors test, with ATCSs, 97-17, 03-14, 03-20
...spiral aftereffect, 64-9, 64-10, 64-17, 68-10, 69-15, 71-31
...stain for dieldrin and endrin, 66-26
...State Trait Anxiety Inventory, 72-23, 76-13, 80-14, 81-5, 89-7, 91-8
...Stroop test, 71-7, 72-14
...supervisory, air traffic control, 92-16
...system for combustion toxicology, 77-9
...vestibular during physical exams, 75-4
...video game experience, 97-4

Tobacco

...effects on aviation safety, 80-11, 83-4

Tolerance

...brain, to concussion, 71-13, 74-4
...cold stress in dogs, 87-8
...decompression for SST, 70-12
...face, to impact, 65-20, 66-12, 66-40
...flight stresses, 62-6, 81-2
...free-fall impacts, 63-15
...heat for rats and mice, 86-8
...heat stress in dogs, 77-8, 81-11, 84-5, 87-8
...hot environments, 70-22
...hypoxia, propranolol effects, 79-10, 80-10
...impacts in water, 65-12, 68-19
...intercontinental flights, 65-16, 65-28, 65-29, 65-30
...orthostatic, 63-34, 82-3, 82-4., 92-19
....+Gz, 79-8, 81-2
...prediction for thermal environments, 71-4
...vertical impact, 62-19
...work at altitudes, 82-3

Toxicology

...beta blocker, forensic analyses and differentiation, 04-15, 05-10
...butalbital, forensic analysis, 00-29
...cocaine and its metabolites, post mortem analyses, 03-23, 03-24
...carbon monoxide, 89-4, 93-7, 94-7, 94-18, 98-21, 00-9, 05-9
...combustion products of cabin materials, 77-9, 85-5, 86-1, 86-3, 86-5, 89-4, 90-15, 90-16, 91-17, 93-7, 93-8
...DNA, detection of ethanol-producing microorganisms in postmortem samples, 00-16
 –identification of forensic specimens, 06-14
 –profiling, quality assurance in forensic, 98-18, 99-14
...enantiomeric analysis of ephedrines and norephedrines, 05-8
...fatal aircraft accident findings, 78-31, 80-11, 82-15, 92-23, 92-24, 94-14, 97-14, 98-5, 99-29, 03-7, 03-22, 03-23, 05-9, 05-20, 06-3, 06-5, 06-12
...gene expression profiles, maintenance after blood storage, 04-1
...glucose levels, abnormal, 00-22
...hydrogen cyanide, 93-8, 94-7, 94-18, 05-9
...hydrogen sulfide, 00-34
...interpretation of carboxyhemoglobin and cyanide concentrations, 05-9
...melatonin, 98-10
...metabolites, 95-26, 97-14

...methamphetamines, 03-22
...methodology, single extraction urine screening, 96-17
  –determination of poppy seed consumption vs. poppy seed use, 05-11
  –enantiomeric analysis of ephedrines and norephedrines, 05-8
  –interpretation of carboxyhemoglobin and cyanide concentrations, 05-9
  –simultaneous quantification of atenolol, metoprolol, and propranolol, 05-10
...opiate use, postmortem determination, 5-11
...ozone toxicity, 80-16, 89-13
...postmortem ethanol analysis, internal standard, 98-5
  –accurate assignment of ethanol origin postmortem, 04-4
  –preservation of tissue samples, 04-4
...postmortem medication findings and pilot medical history, 06-12
...proficiency testing, 99-11
...quality assurance and quality control, 99-11, 99-14, 99-15, 99-29, 03-18, 04-1, 04-4, 04-13, 04-15, 06-14
...RNA isolation from peripheral blood cells, protocol validation, 04-1
...selective serotonin reuptake inhibitors (SSRIs), 03-7
...sildenafil (Viagra), method for detecting in postmortem samples, 00-20, 06-3
...thermal degradation of engine oils, 83-12
...time to incapacitation, 89-4, 93-7, 93-8, 94-7
...Vardenafil (Levitra), method for detecting in postmortem samples, 06-17

Training

...air traffic controllers, 78-10, 79-3, 79-18, 80-5, 80-15, 82-2, 83-9, 84-6, 88-3, 89-6, 89-7, 91-9, 91-18, 94-8, 95-16, 97-15, 98-8, 98-22, 98-23, 99-16, 00-12, 04-21
...aviation medical examiners, 84-7
...biographical factors in ATCS success, 83-6, 84-6
...correlates of satisfaction with, 91-9
...crew resource management, flight inspector aircrew, 96-24
...devices, 96-6
...disorientation familiarization, 70-17, 77-24
...diversity awareness, 95-10
...flight, PC-based training, 94-25, 95-6, 96-8, 97-11, 03-3
...flight instructors, 96-3
...flight physiology, need for, 91-13, 03-10
...flight service station, 86-6, 91-4
...judgment training for pilots, 87-6, 98-6
...maintenance personnel, 91-16, 93-5, 95-14, 95-31, 96-2
...management training, effectiveness of, 75-9, 78-32
...needs for managers, 90-2
...personality factor in ATC, 93-4
...physiological, 10-year chamber experience, 77-4
...reception of distorted speech, 73-13
...resource management, controller/crew, 95-21
...safety seminars for pilots, evaluation, 97-16, 99-7
...situation awareness, 94-27
...stress in pilot training, 67-15, 69-12, 76-2
...supervisory, air traffic control, 92-16
...teamwork, 99-24, 00-24
...test fairness, 79-3, 96-8, 99-16
...tracking performance during successive approaches, 72-9
...transfer from simulation, 69-24, 94-25, 95-6
...water survival programs, analysis, 98-19

Translations

...aviation medicine, general, 64-16, 65-17, 66-2, 68-7, 71-5, 72-16, 73-19, 76-4, 81-4
...color vision tests, 67-8
...nystagmus and vestibular function, Tech. Pub. #1, 1963

Turbulence

...effects of severe weather flying, 66-41
...injuries, cabin safety data bank, 79-23, 82-8

Vertigo

...Coriolis stimulation, 67-19
...flicker, 66-39
...illumination during angular deceleration, 68-28
...in-flight case with unconsciousness, 63-21
...production by spiral aftereffect, 64-9, 64-10, 64-17

Vestibular function

...adaptation, 66-37, 67-6, 67-7, 67-12, 67-19, 69-20, 74-3
...alcohol effects, 71-6, 71-16, 71-20, 71-34, 71-39, 72-34, 79-9
...arousal effects, 62-17, 63-29
...caloric habituation, 63-14, 64-14, 65-18, 67-2
...dextroamphetamine and secobarbital effects, 73-17
...habituation to rotation, 63-13, 65-24, 68-2
...motion sickness susceptibility, 76-14
...rotation device, 64-15
...secondary, tertiary, and inverted primary nystagmus, 63-3
...sleep loss effects, 86-9
...tests during physical examinations, 75-4
...translation of reports, Tech. Pub. #1, 64-16, 65-17, 66-2, 72-16, 73-19

Part III: Subject Index

Vibration

...bibliography, 63-30

Video games

...experience and air traffic scenario test score, 97-4

Vigilance

...eye blink rate and fatigue, 94-17, 94-26, 96-9, 99-28
...hypoxia effects, 71-11
...napping and ATC performance, 00-10
...psychophysiological indices, 99-28
...simulated ATC tasks, 77-18, 78-11, 80-17, 94-6, 94-26, 95-23

Vision

...acuity, pilots in midair collisions, 75-5
...age and binocular fusion time, 66-35
   ...aircraft maintenance inspectors, visual standards and tests, 05-21
...alcohol effects, 78-2, 79-15
...anticollision lights, 66-39, 70-9, 70-15, 71-42, 72-8
...aphakia, accident risk assessment, 95-11
   –incidence in airmen, 91-14, 92-14, 93-11
...artificial lens implants, 92-14, 93-11
...atropine and Phosdrin effects, 73-4
...bifocal effects on radar monitoring, 82-16
...bright lights and visual disturbances during nighttime flight operations, 06-28
...Broca-Sulzer phenomenon, 68-27
...chart readability, 77-13, 78-17
...color, diagnostic tests, 67-8, 71-27, 71-32, 73-18, 75-1, 93-16, 93-17, 95-13, 96-22, 04-10, 04-14
...color perception and ATCS job performance, 83-11, 85-7, 90-3, 92-6, 92-28, 92-29, 04-10, 04-14, 06-2, 06-6, 06-11, 06-15, 06-22
...contact lenses in an airline accident, 00-18
   –in certification, 90-10, 00-18
...cues for approach and landing, 79-4, 79-25, 81-6, 82-6
...deficiencies in accident airmen, 81-14, 83-18, 93-11
...disorientation, 69-23, 70-2
...drug and pesticide effects on visual reflexes, 79-15
...fatigue effects on binocular fusion time, 69-1
...fixation effects on nystagmus, 67-12
...gender differences in refractive surgery, 00-23
...glare, 94-15, 03-6
...glaucoma, visual field and altitude, 91-1
...illusions, 70-2, 71-22, 77-12, 78-15
...instrument readability by senior pilots, 77-2, 77-7
...laser illumination effects, 03-12, 04-9, 06-23
...light adaptation device, 66-38
...matching flash loudness and brightness, 67-16
...monitoring performance on simulated radar task, 80-17, 81-12, 82-16, 90-3, 94-17, 94-26, 96-9
...occupational vision, 96-12, 96-27
...ophthalmic lenses for air traffic controllers, 96-12, 96-27
...perception of depth, 63-10, 63-28, 67-20
...perception of size and distance, 62-15, 64-13, 65-11, 66-22, 66-24, 67-18
...perception of spatial extent, 63-20
...peripheral visual cues, 68-11, 68-12, 68-22
...photorefractive keratectomy, 98-25
...presbyopic individuals, 77-14
...propeller paint schemes conspicuity, 78-29
...reaction time, flash luminance and brightness, 67-24
...radial keratectomy, 98-25, 06-9
...radial keratotomy, 99-6, 00-19, 06-9
...readability of emergency signs in smoke, 79-22, 80-13, 81-7
...refractive surgery, 99-6, 00-19, 00-23, 06-9
...restrictions and pilot demographics, 04-6
...search performance with radar sweepline, 79-12
...smoke-protective goggles, 76-5, 78-41, 83-14
...spiral aftereffect, 64-9, 64-10, 64-17, 68-10, 69-15, 71-31
...stimulation during angular deceleration, 68-28
...sunscreen materials effects, 78-28
...test for monitoring and scanning, 92-12, 94-8
...two-flash thresholds, 68-20, 70-15, 71-42
...X-Chrom lens to improve color vision, 78-22

Warning signals

...blink amplitudes and attention, 97-10, 99-8
...color and flashing radar targets, 90-3
...pilot hearing thresholds, 05-12

Water survival

...ditching, factors in passenger flow rates, 04-12
...flotation, use of seat cushion, 95-20
...life preserver evaluations, 85-11, 03-9
...training programs, analysis, 98-19

Weight

...accident rate relation to body weight, 70-18
...ATCS population, changes in, 71-19, 72-20
...errors in stated estimates, 73-10
...third-class certificate holders, changes in, 72-26

Work

...age and retirement of air traffic controllers, 05-6, 05-22
...age effects on tolerance, 63-33
...alcohol effects, 82-3
...altitude effects on tolerance, 63-33, 82-3

...anxiety, relation to workload in ATCSs, 73-15, 77-23, 80-14, 81-5
...blood pressure effects, 66-36
...capacity, after myocardial infarction, 64-2, 66-17, 66-21
  –of ATCS students, 71-8
  –related to age, 63-18
  –with step test, 64-3
...communication, and controller workload, 01-8
...distractibility with monotony, 72-25
...domestic-based stress, effects on work environment, 00-32
...drug effects on performance, 63-12, 63-34
...energy cost on treadmill, 62-5
...fitness, field test for, 63-6
...human tolerance, 62-6
...measurement, of air traffic controller workload, 98-15, 05-16, 06-29
  –of information complexity in automation design, 04-17
  –of pilot workload, 77-15, 81-13
...monotonous task performance correlates, 73-14
...motivation of ATCS, 73-2
...organizational climate, ATC, 04-23,
  –FAA, 98-24, 03-11, 04-22, 04-23, 05-13, 06-30
  –FSS, 97-12
...passenger workload and protective breathing requirements, 87-2
...safety climate, 97-8, 99-19
...shift rotation effects, 65-5, 65-6, 81-4, 82-17, 83-17, 85-2, 86-2, 06-13
...shiftwork and performance, 97-25, 99-2, 00-10
...sickle cell trait effects, 80-20
...strength and endurance of female pilots, 72-27, 73-23
...strength of flight attendants, 75-13
...thermal balance in heat and cold, 66-23, 68-13
...workload effects, on complex performance, 83-15
  –flight progress strips, 98-26

www.ingramcontent.com/pod-product-compliance
Lightning Source LLC
Chambersburg PA
CBHW081829170526
45167CB00007B/2754